SHUT YOUR M   AND OPEN WIDE

DR ELMAR JUNG

● ● ●

dot dot dot publishing

dot dot dot publishing

• • •

edge-of-your-seat books

ADVISORY NOTE

Shut Your Mouth and Open Wide is for informational purposes only. The theories and practices explained are based on the personal opinion of the author.

The contents of the book are based on scientific literature and the experience of the author. The contents of this book do not reflect mainstream opinion of either medicine or dentistry—at least, not yet.

Nothing in this book is intended to diagnose or treat any disease or condition. It is neither medical nor dental advice, nor should it be construed as such.

Always seek the opinion of the relevant qualified health professional before making any changes to your diet, prescription drug use, lifestyle, exercise activities or before undergoing any dental procedure.

CONTENTS

INTRODUCTION

A terrifying sound no parent wants to hear.

A child screaming out of fear, out of sheer terror.

First, he hit her. Then he choked her. Then he started ripping out one tooth after the other. She was only six years old. She was writhing, screaming.

He would not stop.

Only after seven of her tiny front teeth were pulled did it come to an end.

Horror in the dentist chair. All done without anaesthetic.

Reports were written. Complaints filed, tears shed. But the police did not listen. They even denied the existence of the reports. No investigation was launched.

The sadistic torturer made almost four million dollars in just five years with his appalling, criminal, deeply disturbing and abusive dentistry.

He traumatised children for life. He was a parent's worst nightmare.

The government funded every single tooth he extracted or treated. He profited by performing fraudulent, unnecessary treatments on the healthy teeth of the young, the most vulnerable.

Sixteen crowns on a three-year-old child!

He even wore scary costumes and threatened children by telling them, "Your mom will die if you tell her what happened."

Only when one mum made the bold move to record her daughter's dental treatment was this charlatan exposed.

His crimes in the dental chair were revealed and his case caught fire. A wildfire. An online frenzy on Facebook. It was unbelievable how many children he had terrorised. Then the lawsuits started coming in.

Dr. Howard Schneider from Florida is an example of the worst that could happen in dentistry.

This is an extreme example of very real and very bad dentistry. A nightmare feared by parents and dental patients alike. Thankfully, it is very rare.

However, there is another form of dentistry, less dramatic, subtler and more pervasive. Yet its impact on us and our lives can be just as brutal. It is called *Toxic Dentistry*, and in this book you will:

- Learn about the hidden toxins in dentistry and the threat they pose to you and your family.
- Debunk the myth that your teeth are just for chewing. Your overall health depends on a healthy mouth.
- Explore the interaction between your teeth and your emotional state, recognising how this can influence your oral health.
- Understand why nutrition is fundamental for optimal dental health and overall well-being.
- Discover what you can do to improve your dental health and how to maintain it for life.

You may find some of the information in this book strange and unfamiliar. However, empirical evidence and documented research strongly supports this approach.

Stay curious and keep an open mind.

You'll start to understand that everything in your body is interconnected.

Like a hologram, every cell holds the information of your entire body. Nothing in us is wasted or useless. It is just that we do not fully understand the human body, yet.

You will explore the connection that your teeth have with other parts of your body such as organs, joints, vertebrae, sensory organs and many more. We call this the tooth-body connection.

Examples drawn from more than twenty-five years of my dental experience highlight patients' very real and pressing challenges and how they benefitted from appropriate dental treatment.

Holistic dentists do much more than just drill, fill and bill. They actively remove obstacles from patients' mouths which frequently have a knock-on effect on their overall health symptoms.

This book is your essential starting point as you create optimal health for you and your loved ones.

So now, it is time to…

Shut Your Mouth and Open Wide

DENTISTRY
THE BASICS

1. Toxins

Every day toxins are slowly killing you.

Toxins are everywhere. Toxins surround you, toxins are in you. Toxins are suffocating you with every breath you take.

You drink toxins with every sip of water. You ingest toxins with your food. Your home is saturated in toxins.

One of the most pernicious ways of getting toxins in your body is a simple trip to your dentist.

Just for a moment, imagine your next dental treatment. You are a bit nervous. You feel the numbness from the anaesthetic. The dentist drills away the decay. Then you open wide again. He is about to place material into your tooth to fill the hole.

Your eyes are looking around and in the very angle of your view you see this package with a skull-and-crossbones warning sign printed on it—extreme danger! Your heart beats faster. *Impossible!* The first thought which shoots through your confused mind. *He wouldn't do that. NO!*

But he does, he comes closer with the filling material and closer still. You jump off the chair and you run, run fast, run away.

As you run. You think, *Hang on! THEY wouldn't allow this. Allow poison? Poison my mouth. Poison my teeth. My gums. My bones. My whole body. They ban poison. Ban it from the start. They want you healthy. Don't they?*

And as you think this, your pace slows, *Why are people getting sicker and sicker? Why are billions invested in medical research, yet still no cures are found for chronic dis-eases and cancer or even for supposedly simple things like tooth decay?*

What does dentistry have to do with all of this? Dentistry can be dark, dangerous and harmful. And it is so widespread it even has its own name—*Toxic Dentistry*.

In dentistry we come across quite a few potentially toxic materials. The main ones are mercury amalgam fillings, root canal fillings and fluorides. There is also other toxic bacterial waste from gum disease, root canal-treated teeth and necrotic bone infections.

Bluntly, dentistry uses the most toxic treatments in medicine, apart from chemotherapy and radiation.

Despite overwhelming proof, devastated lives and the unimaginable suffering of affected people, the official story still claims that these materials and treatments are safe for us.

We also read and hear similar statements from so-called experts and the industry's advocates that fluoride prevents tooth decay and jawbone cavitations don't exist.

What has to happen for these health-threatening poisons to disappear from the world of dentistry?

2. Mercury Amalgam

Mercury amalgam is the filling material they place into your mouth. Dental amalgam is made from mercury, silver, tin, zinc and copper. In dentistry they dare to call it silver amalgam, to give it a healthier name.

Is it bad, ugly, dark, dangerous and poisonous, or the best invention in dentistry since sliced bread? Does the fact that it is affordable, easy to use and long-lasting make it attractive to the dental industry?

Mercury, facts and fiction!

Can you honestly say you know the facts from the fiction when it comes to mercury?

Is mercury really that toxic or are some health fanatics just overreacting? Mercury has been used in dentistry for more than 150 years. Surely it cannot be that toxic or *they* would have stopped its use a long time ago. Wouldn't they?

So, it is time to decide what comes closest to the truth and what is myth. The facts can't be easily dismissed. However, knowing the facts makes it easier to separate them from the lies.

The facts:

Amalgam consists of more than 50% mercury. Mercury is a neurotoxin; therefore, amalgam fillings are neurotoxins.

Mercury is leaking out from each and every filling twenty-four hours a day, seven days a week.

Mercury amalgam fillings are the most toxic dental material still in use.

If you chew, drink a hot drink, grind your teeth or have different metals in your mouth, the amount of mercury released increases far beyond the maximum allowance at your workplace.

Mercury-related symptoms are extensive.

Mercury intoxication symptoms are exhibited neurologically, emotionally and dermatologically: metallic taste, mood swings, irritability, headaches, insomnia, hyperactivity, increased sweating, muscle twitching, anxiety, tremors, learning difficulties, skin problems, muscle weakness and chronic candida.

Mercury accumulates mainly in your kidneys, spleen, liver, bones, stomach, brain, spine, thyroid and fatty tissues.

By accumulating in the thyroid, mercury reduces the thyroid's capacity to provide sufficient energy for the adrenals. Poor thyroid function means poor adrenal function.

Mercury also plays a role in diseases of the nervous system such as multiple sclerosis, Alzheimer's, Parkinson's, and amyotrophic lateral sclerosis as well as in chronic fatigue syndrome.

Mercury makes bacteria resistant to antibiotics and can trigger periodontal disease. Mercury affects hormone production, blocks enzymes and compromises the immune system.

Pregnant women detoxify themselves of their mercury load directly into their unborn child via the umbilical cord. Whilst breastfeeding the mercury loads transfer via the mother's milk.

A single dose of mercury (the amount of a single inhalation) takes one to two months to be eliminated from your body. As you inhale about 17,000 times a day, it is clear that mercury will build up in your body. To eliminate a fraction of the mercury you have accumulated in your brain can take many years or even decades.

Just removing the toxic mercury fillings will not remove the toxic load from your organs. There is no such thing as a safe level of mercury in the human body. *The World Health Organisation* states that mercury from fillings is a significant source of mercury burden in the body.

When removed from your mouth, any amalgam scrap has to be disposed as hazardous waste. It appears that your mouth is believed to be the only safe place to keep mercury.

Mercury is being phased out in almost every industrial and medical context across the EU to severely reduce its environmental contamination.

Now ask yourself again, what is fact and what is fiction about mercury amalgam fillings?

3. Root Canal

Imagine for a moment you are stuck in a cave. A dark, underground hole. No light, no air, no sounds. You cannot see or hear a thing. Much worse, you cannot breathe.

With the last vestiges of air in your lungs you have to feel your way through a daunting labyrinth of tiny little tunnels to reach the main chamber. Only there will you get the desperately needed oxygen in order to survive. Will you make it?

Anaerobic bacteria thrive on the absence of oxygen. They appreciate the darkness. They are full of joy; welcoming the absence of oxygen because they hate it. Oxygen kills them.

Bacteria float easily in these tiny little tunnels. It is like a vacation for them. Floating along in shorts and cossies on lazy rivers with rubber rings, giggling away in these oxygen-free tunnels, having the time of their lives whilst pooping in your mouth!

They are grateful for their tiny size because they know that nothing, no liquid nor detergent, not even oxygen, is capable of reaching their sanctuary.

They feel pampered and very, very safe.

Now, from a tooth-saving point of view, a root canal treatment seems to be the perfect choice for the patient. However, when you look more closely at what happens when a root canal is performed, it shines a whole different light on the procedure.

If your big toe was to develop gangrene, would your GP recommend removing the nerves, blood and lymph vessels and sticking some pins in the toe to save it? Very unlikely.

They are more likely to recommend removing the toe in order to prevent the infection from spreading.

Your tooth is a living organ just like your toe. Does a root canal treatment deal with the core infection challenge?

Even if you would consider this treatment plausible, it is impossible to completely clean the entire tooth of these bacteria because the tooth has two to three miles of tiny microscopically small channels.

No treatments are capable of accessing these tiny channels. And this is where bacteria hide and excrete their toxic waste into your body.

Once in your bloodstream, these toxins can spread all over your body and cause harm to susceptible organs, joints and muscle tissues.

4. Osteonecrosis Infection

His agony, his suffering started slowly, years ago. He hardly remembers when.

"No hope," they said.

They gave up on him. He gave up on himself, almost.

Always in pain. Always in bed. Always uncomfortable. For years.

In pain, in lots of pain, unbearable pain. His entire body in pain. Pain with every move. Pain with every thought. And drained of energy, exhausted. His memory took a hit too.

Years of shoulder and arm pain, back problems, rheumatic problems, migraines, headaches, chronic fatigue, skin problems, heart disease, facial, joint, nerve and muscle pain.

Thousands of pounds spent on hundreds of tests, without getting any closer to the cause. Numerous treatments completed and medications swallowed, all without getting any better.

"It is all in your head." That's what they told him. And they were right. It was the hole in his jawbone. The cause of years of suffering!

Not easily detected on most X-rays, these holes are masters at hiding. Toxic infection in your jawbone. Another minefield in dentistry where opinions are at war with the facts.

Many dentists, let alone patients, haven't even heard of them. Many dentists who have heard of them do not believe they exist.

But a small and growing number of dental colleagues know these holes DO exist. They have seen them, they have treated them and they have witnessed some of the most miraculous and positive effects on their patients' health.

Osteonecrosis infection has many names: cavitation, Ratner-bone lesion, fatty-degenerative osteolysis jawbone (Fdoj), cavitational osteonecrosis, chronic osteomyelitis jawbone cavitation and silent inflammation, etc.

If undetected and untreated it can become a serious health threat.

These holes develop mainly after a tooth extraction, especially after wisdom tooth extraction. A trauma such as a blow to the face can also be the reason for developing a necrotic bone infection.

The reason they appear is either because the extraction site has not been cleaned out thoroughly, something intervened with the healing process, or the body was simply too exhausted to heal properly.

Under normal circumstances these holes do not cause any local symptoms, not even pain, which makes it difficult to look for them in the first place, simply because the patient does not complain about any symptoms in this area.

If they cause pain, they are called NICO-lesions (Neuralgia-Inducing-Cavitational-Osteonecrosis).

All osteonecrosis infections are ideal hiding places for bacteria which live without oxygen. They are breeding grounds for chronic diseases due to the toxic waste the bacteria produce.

Similar to root canaled teeth, the osteonecrosis appears like a gangrene in the bone and the toxic waste produced by the bacteria can cause harm in other parts of your body, seemingly unrelated to the infected area.

5. Implants

The nightmare began only hours after she had the new tooth fitted.

"No big deal," they had told her. "Implants in a day. Tooth out. Implant in."

She always wanted the ugly black tooth out and was very happy to have it done in less than an hour.

But where did that weird metallic taste come from all of a sudden? And the tingling in her lip, teeth and chin? And why was it still bleeding?

A few days later she did not even make it out of bed. Her underlying chronic fatigue took over. Her aches and pains caused her massive frustration. It drove her crazy.

Can toxic dentistry be so powerful that it causes such havoc to people who suffer from underlying health issues? Or even worse, can toxic dentistry become the trigger to develop chronic diseases in the first place?

But her friend had the same treatment with more implants. And she was absolutely fine after the procedure and remained so years after the treatment.

"Why me, again?" She complained.

When implants were developed in the 1950s they came as a godsend for toothless patients. Finally, they were capable of chewing their food properly again and the uncomfortable palate-covering, taste-inhibiting and confidence-reducing smelly dentures could finally be a thing of the past.

Nowadays, the desire for a perfect set of teeth and a Hollywood smile seems to be far more important than any health concern raised.

It also seems that many dentists have found their Holy Grail and are placing implants left, right and centre into every single gap they discover. It is a billion-dollar industry, and everyone wants a piece of it.

A research engineer mentioned that most implants never fully integrate into the bone. "An integration of 60% already counts as success, but is only reached by a very few. The average integration of an implant into the bone is more like 40%," he said. "And X-rays do not show the real situation."

13 | AND OPEN WIDE

This corresponds with the experience of many holistic dentists when taking out implants. Many implants can be unscrewed rather easily, which means there has been no bone integration at all.

Often the bone holding the implant is infected and soft. Therefore, many patients lose a lot of bone when having these areas cleaned out.

The evaluation and indication for placing implants has to be very thorough. I would be wary of recommending implants to patients with underlying immune-system compromising diseases.

If you opt for implants, opt for metal-free, zirconium oxide implants.

6. FLUORIDES

Horror! Big time!

Eight-year-old Emily stands before her mirror looking at her reflection, staring at her teeth. Curiously she starts to examine her new permanent teeth. The incisors are just making their way through the gum.

Gazing more closely into the mirror she gets absorbed by the discolouring of these teeth.

Some of them are brown and have tiny white spots. Now she realises those disgusting patches are hers. Screaming in horror, she runs to her mum.

What has happened to her teeth?

Those blemishes, how horrible they look, really unhealthy. It is as if she had not brushed her teeth properly. They look almost as if her teeth are decaying, hideous, repulsive.

What will her friends at school think? With her birthday party looming what will her relatives think of her? Her teeth look so ugly!

Emily starts to feel the panic creeping up her spine. Her mum has to comfort her.

How will she look in photos? She cannot show her beautiful smile anymore, not now anyway. She can hardly put her hand in front of her mouth. People will grimace in terror when they see her smiling with all these dirty looking specks on the teeth.

If you were at an important event and need to be smiling, yet you have these awful brown and white spots on your teeth, how would you feel?

Despite religiously brushing, flossing, and water flossing! You cannot believe it, you dare not look in the mirror! That's what other people see when they talk with you. Better not talk to anyone anymore.

How to get it sorted? Why did it happen?

Fluorosis.

In other words, over-fluoridation!

The cause of the decayed-looking teeth is the chemical that is advertised to *prevent* tooth decay from happening.

The opinions on the risks and benefits of water fluoridation, fluoride in toothpastes, tablets, mouthwashes, dental filling materials or salt vary considerably.

However, looking at the facts again, makes it very easy to establish that there is little benefit to support its use and this benefit rests 100% with the companies who sell it to you.

The fluoride that may be put in the water supply is forced medication in unmeasured amounts. Even the fluoride in toothpaste lacks sound and unflawed evidence from studies for its marketed properties.

Only American communities and countries under strong American influence persist in the practice.

Denmark, Holland, Sweden, China, Russia, Austria and Belgium, India and Hungary have banned it. Other countries have restricted its use.

About 10% of the UK population (mainly in the Midlands and North East) have their water fluoridated. In the US around 170 million people receive this kind of medication.

Tooth decay is not a fluoride-lacking disease. Fluoride does not reduce tooth decay.

There is evidence that excess fluoride is responsible for problems such as brittle bone, osteoporosis and even osteosarcomas, a deadly bone cancer of young males.

Your thyroid suffers badly from fluoride accumulation because fluoride mimics iodine and acts as a hormone disruptor, causing thyroid cell death, thyroid inflammation and autoimmune diseases like Hashimoto's amongst many other problems.

Babies' brains and hormonal systems also suffer from excess fluoridation.

Excess fluoride increases genetic damage, hip fractures and infertility.

Adding fluoride to the water supply to prevent tooth decay is as sensible as adding sun cream to the water supply to prevent sun burn.

She should look more carefully where she is going. The little rocks are everywhere. What will happen, will happen.

She hit her toe on that damned, jagged little rock. Now her toe is swollen. It is red. It is hot. It hurts like hell.

She can feel her blood pulsing in her toe. She knows it, she feels it, she can almost hear her toe screaming at her, "I caught an infection."

Lots of people think bugs are bad. They think germs are grim, bacteria do harm, are evil. They think bacteria can kill and that you have to kill them first. They think you need strong antibiotics to crush them, to show them who is boss, to set an example, warn them off. And they think you have to do it quickly. You have to be the winner. You have to survive.

Bacteria are all around you. In the air you breathe, the water you drink, the food you eat and in your home.

They are on your skin, in your nose, in your lungs, in your stomach, in your intestines. You exchange them with every kiss or bodily interaction.

Bacteria are everywhere. You are living in a bacterial world.

People think that bacteria do so much harm, that they cause so many diseases and so much pain. They ruin people's lives. We have to destroy them, wreck their lives, beat them, make them extinct. Live a life without bacteria.

But look again! Think again! What do bacteria do? A visit to your mouth will give you an idea.

Your mouth offers the perfect climate for bacteria to live and grow because it is moist and warm. But not everybody suffers from tooth decay or gum disease.

Without bacteria we wouldn't be alive.

Bacteria are opportunistic, they use what is given to them. They get away with what they can. They are clever, very clever! Why do you think so many antibiotics do not work anymore?

Obviously, there are those bacteria or viruses which are potentially harmful such as Salmonella or Epstein-Barr. And there are also many people living happy lives without symptoms, despite having these bacteria or viruses in their body.

So, we have to get much better at understanding this almost invisible world. The fear of bacteria and some people's almost insane drive for cleanliness, has made the situation worse rather than better.

Especially regarding our children who are over-protected. They do not get in contact with dirt anymore and therefore miss out on building their natural immune system.

What if bacteria, viruses and fungi are Nature's way of helping us repair and heal the body? What if bad nutrition, lack of sleep, exercise or sunshine are the reasons for disease?

Or stress and fear? Or the shock of an event? Or the dental materials in your mouth?

8. Tooth Decay

You are horrified. You just looked in the mirror. It is not the tired-looking eyes that you notice.

Something else is grimacing at you. A substantial, black, ugly hole on your lower-left first molar. That must have grown overnight. It definitely was not there when you had a look a few days ago. Your day is totally ruined. You are devastated.

Tooth decay. A massive nightmare.

You will have to call your best friend to drag you to the dentist. You will never make it on your own. *Dentist? Oh no!*

You know exactly what this means. It will start with being told off for not coming in earlier. Then pain. Pain when the dentist digs into your tooth, gives you the injection, and even more pain when the dentist drills too quickly.

Pain is all you can think about. And that disgusting smell of burning bone and that terrible taste of whatever in God's name it is.

The big question however is, "Can she save the tooth?"

The next thing you remember is waking up drenched in sweat, running to the bathroom, looking in the mirror. The black hole has miraculously disappeared. Thank God, it really was only just a nightmare.

Why do teeth decay despite them being the hardest substance in your body? It must be a very aggressive process to destroy such incredibly resistant material.

Do not listen to the story of bacteria being the culprit of tooth decay or the lack of fluoride being responsible for it. It is not even your oral hygiene.

The cause for tooth decay happens to lie somewhere totally different. It is rooted in your diet, your lifestyle. This has been proven true over centuries by tribes who have never been in contact with our Western diet, who do not suffer tooth decay and often do not even have a word for tooth decay or gum disease.

You are unlikely to develop tooth decay, in fact any kind of disease, if you strive for a healthy diet, exercise sufficiently, get a good night's sleep, know how to balance your stress levels and your emotions and get enough sunlight.

Once you know tooth decay has hit you, you have to realise that something is fundamentally wrong inside your body.

Tooth decay is not a localised problem. Tooth decay, like any other dis-ease, is your body's way of telling you that you are out of balance.

9. GUM DISEASE

Blood everywhere. Your toothbrush soaked in blood, the sink covered in blood and your mouth full of it. Where does all that blood come from? You did not brush too hard, nor did you eat something that could have caused this much blood. How did it get so bad?

A few weeks ago, you saw a tiny sprinkle of blood on your brand-new toothbrush when cleaning the upper-left front teeth. *That happened before,* you tell yourself, *it will also disappear like before.*

But not this time. This time it stayed. And it got worse. Much worse. Now you are looking at a real mess. Blood everywhere.

Not only do you taste and smell blood, you also feel something is not quite right. Something is going on with one of your teeth up there on the left.

Oh no! You freeze; the tooth is moving. How can a tooth move? Is it not supposed to be fixed in the bone? But this one is definitely mobile!

And this time it is for real. Not just a bad dream. This tooth actually moves, and it hurts, and there is blood everywhere. Now you have to act. And act fast. *Phone the dentist now!*

Gum disease, like tooth decay, is not a mysterious condition that strikes at random or without warning.

Like any other disease it develops because a disturbed and unbalanced environment offers micro-organisms the opportunity to flourish.

In a healthy mouth and a healthy body, bacteria are usually free-floating and not harmful, or at least can be kept in check.

However, gum disease nowadays is the most common disease affecting the majority of adults.

It is the number one reason why people lose their teeth. It is a very serious infection which is connected to other diseases such as heart attacks, diabetes, arthritis, cardio-vascular disease, and arteriosclerosis. It can even affect pregnancy and fertility.

Mainstream medicine nowadays admits the connection between this oral problem and its effects on other organs and on a patient's overall health.

If you suffer from gum disease your saliva is most likely acidic.

There are obvious contributing factors like smoking, amalgam fillings, poorly done dentistry, mouth breathing, incorrect bite, hormonal imbalances or oral contraceptives. All of which help pave the way for gum disease.

As with tooth decay and any other so-called local disease, it is just showing you the tip of the iceberg: you have to dig deeper to get to the source.

When suffering from gum disease or any kind of infectious disease, replace your toothbrush weekly.

Even if you have a healthy diet and clean your teeth properly, you will have tens of thousands of bacteria living on each tooth surface. Those with less than ideal diets and poor oral hygiene will have 100 to 1000 times more.

As long as your internal ecosystem is balanced, bacteria live in harmony with you.

10. TOOTHACHE

It hits you like lightning. It hits you at the worst time. It hits you right out of the blue in your face, in your mouth, in your tooth.

Toothache is, without doubt, a most unpleasant experience. We avoid it like the plague.

It is something you might wish on your ex, on your worst enemy or even your dentist.

It is a dull ache that turns into an electric jolt when you bite down on the tooth.

However, it has the positive virtue of concentrating your attention, which you might have wasted elsewhere, to a very narrow point inside of you—your tooth, which is screaming out, "Help me!"

You have barely felt the first sting, endured the familiar wincing and you have already forgotten the world around you: looming dinner date, tax returns, what's on TV. Money concerns or job challenges suddenly become null and void. Even friends seem to be forgotten.

There is only one thing that holds your attention, that is of importance. The one thing that is lurking in your tooth. And you want to get rid of it *now*, even if it means having the tooth removed. Anything is better than this excruciating pain.

Very few types of pain can make your life such a constant misery as toothache. Only if you have experienced this kind of pain will you understand.

However, toothache is merely the body's warning signal that something is not going according to plan. The root cause does not even have to be where the pain is. The pain could merely be the flashing light to get your attention for a serious problem elsewhere in your body.

Pain, from a more holistic point of view, is always a sign that the energy flow is interrupted or blocked. Therefore, toothache is a symptom which needs further investigation.

Throbbing pain for example can indicate an infected pulp, a periodontal abscess or a healing problem after surgery.

If you experience an ache in your mouth for more than a few days, an appointment with your dentist should be the first call of action. He will examine your mouth and distinguish where the pain stems from and also recommend the appropriate treatment.

11. STRUCTURE AND YOUR BITE

It hurts. It hurts a lot! He wishes he had listened to his parents. But now it is too late for regrets. Now it has already happened. No way to turn back time.

The oak tree was just too intriguing. His parents had gone out with some friends and he thought this time he could do it on his own. The garden was all his.

"Owwwaah!" It really hurts. He thought he was so clever. He had prepared everything. But then he lost his balance and fell off the ladder. Now the leg looks a strange shape. Could it be broken? He wails in agony. The pain is something else. This is a disaster.

The ladder was the problem. No even ground to keep the balance. No solid staves to support the climb. No stability to make it work. It was destined to fail.

Like the ladder, our skeletal system has to be in balance and has to have support and stability. Without this harmony between balance, support and stability it will not function properly.

Few people realise that teeth are such an important part of the skeletal system. The way your top and bottom teeth fit together is crucial for the balance of your whole body and is a determining factor for the correct posture of your head, shoulders and hips.

Only if the joints match the chewing-system (temporomandibular joint—TMJ) correctly are you free of stress.

If you have a skeletal posture imbalance, your body will create patterns that compensate, either up from the hips or down from the head.

You may not notice any discomfort until your body has reached a point where it can no longer adjust without pain. It is vital that the underlying cause is treated.

If your body is not properly balanced, all dental work to correct the bite will not last long term, unless the work is combined with postural work. The same is true the other way round.

When teeth are not in harmony, tooth grinding can occur and this could harm your teeth; even to the point of breaking them.

When correcting misaligned teeth and jaws, it is crucial to look at the patient's skeletal structure from top to toe.

Especially in children, extracting teeth to create more space is almost always the wrong treatment. It is not too many teeth in the mouth—it is too small a mouth for the teeth!

The jawbones and the arches have to be expanded to create space for all the teeth.

12. Chronic Diseases

In nature everything has a cause. So what cause could a chronic disease have?

Why does anyone suffer from an ongoing skin issue if the epidermis cells are fully renewed after only 30 days? Why do people experience stomach ulcers for more than nine days despite the fact the stomach lining is renewed every nine days?

You have an almost entirely renewed body every eight months. You are a new *you* every eight months.

Is that not fascinating? And daunting.

Because this poses a challenging question. Why do you keep being plagued with diseases longer than those eight months? What are the causes that keep you stuck in your ailment?

Why are food allergies sky rocketing?

Why is the incidence of multiple chemical sensitivity rapidly growing?

Why is autism, heart disease or cancer at an all-time high?

Why are reproductive disorders dramatically increasing?

Why are digestive problems escalating?

Why are more brain tumours found than ever before?

Questions to which mainstream Western medicine fails to provide conclusive answers.

Chronic disease develops whilst you are still able to compensate. However, your bucket fills up over years. Once the bucket is full, once it cannot take any more burden or strain, it will overflow and your capacity to compensate is exhausted.

Could GMOs (Genetically Modified Organisms) trigger chronic diseases?

Will GMOs save mankind from starvation or are they the biggest health threat to humans, animals and plants alike? The fog of misinformation is now lifting, the truth is coming to light and the price for all of this has yet to be paid. Safety studies, are you kidding?

Could your emotions cause your life to disintegrate and chronic disease to develop?

Could intense electromagnetic fields (EMFs) trigger chronic disease due to your ever-increasing use of mobile and cordless phones, Wi-Fi, microwave ovens, smart meters, 5G or any other EMF-emitting device?

Acute disease and chronic disease are two entirely different things. With acute disease, Western medicine comes into its own and excels. With chronic disease it is not that simple.

You do not fall from a tree and get a chronic disease.

There are many different reasons that can cause a chronic disease to develop. By the time you get labelled with a diagnosis, things have already been going wrong for a very long time.

If we only treat symptoms, we will never get rid of the underlying causes and, therefore, will never get rid of the chronic disease itself.

Hardly anyone is in constant optimum health. We are always moving between the range of optimum health and disease. There are times we eat too much, drink too much, have too much emotional stress, lack sleep, do not breathe properly and do not exercise sufficiently. Then our body moves towards dis-ease.

Turning your head towards dentistry you can easily observe that it deals mainly with managing symptoms or, even worse, suppressing them—with root canals or antibiotics—rather than looking at the bigger picture of the ongoing, underlying chronic problem.

Medicine has developed from being an art to a technical endeavour, where symptoms become the enemy rather than the indicator and where disease is seen as something foreign, something bad and wrong. Does nature really make mistakes?

EMOTIONS
MAKING CONNECTIONS

Next time you feel sad have a look at your posture. You will find yourself sitting with your shoulders curving forwards, your head looking to the floor, the corners of your mouth facing downwards and your mind spinning around gloomy thoughts.

Try something now. Stand upright, tighten your arm, legs and stomach muscles, grin enthusiastically, look to the sky or ceiling and say to yourself energetically, "Yes! Yes! Yes! Yes!"

How do you feel?

Your posture affects your emotions and your emotions affect your posture.

This section shows how dental treatments and dental materials can affect emotions and how emotions can influence the health of teeth.

Another routine dental treatment completed. She rinses her mouth.

Suddenly her skin itches. She feels hot. Her tongue starts to swell, her lips too. *What is happening to me?* She starts to panic. Her heart beats faster and faster. Dizziness sets in. She faints, collapses. Her body slides off the dental chair like a rag doll, onto the floor.

Minutes later, she is dead. It's all over!

Killed... by a mouthwash!

Anaphylactic shock. The worst form of allergic reaction.

Allergic reactions are more and more common. Anything can cause an allergic reaction.

You've probably heard of someone or know someone who is allergic to a specific food such as peanuts or shellfish, a specific plant pollen, a material, a medication, an insect bite or some kind of metal such as nickel.

Allergic reactions to amalgam fillings are very rare.

A different form of reaction is the toxic reaction and that is where mercury amalgam scores. The reaction can come suddenly. However, it is more likely it will take a long time. Sometimes it can take years to show any symptoms and most likely the cause of the symptoms remains undetected.

This happens all the time. I hear and see it a lot. The story of how amalgam fillings can turn a patient's well-being into a nightmare. An emotional rollercoaster.

Only a few doctors and dentists seem to know about the neurological and emotional effects mercury amalgam fillings can have on susceptible patients.

However, amalgam is not the only dental material that can trigger emotional reactions. Composite filling materials with their hormone-disrupting ingredients, dead teeth, root canal fillings and implants can also cause emotional upset due to their compromising impact on the body's energy pathways. These pathways, also called meridians, are similar to the body's nerve pathways in that they run through your entire body.

The Chinese discovered the existence of meridians thousands of years ago. However, it wasn't until the 1950s that Dr. Voll and Dr. Kramer discovered that every tooth is connected to specific organs, other parts of the body and also to specific emotional qualities.

Having a gum infection, a root canal-treated tooth, an implant or a filling placed in your mouth can trigger an emotional reaction.

2. Worry and Guilt: The Visit

During the day he worries, whilst his nights are filled with agonising dreams of horror. *What will happen this time?* His mind races. His thoughts of worry, guilt and doubt. He has to stop them. He has to change them. But he can't. He feels guilty for not doing what he was told. The nagging thoughts flood his brain with a tidal wave of emotion. No way of stopping them.

Two more days. Two more very long days. And two more very long sleepless nights until the real nightmare begins. In his mind he has already explored all the terrible things that can happen.

Each morning he dreads the alarm. In 72 hours it will all be over!

For some people the idea of going to the dentist is something inherently paralysing. Something they have avoided for a very long time. But finally, they realise there is no way they can postpone it any further.

Their worry about what will happen in the dental chair and the guilt of having neglected their teeth and gums have led them to this point.

The worry builds up in their mind which creates a fear of the future around the event that may not actually be that bad. It's the story they create in their mind that triggers the worry, not the event itself.

We tend to worry about what we think is beyond our control.

Worry can be overwhelming. It can even lead down the path of mental illness. It can become so extreme that it can lead to substance addiction to help take the worry away.

What we often need is a change to our thinking, a perspective which will help alleviate our mood. However, this is easier said than done. For worriers, it can be beneficial to immerse themselves in an activity they enjoy.

Even if you do have worries about your dental treatment, most of the time your dentist will do all they can to make your visit as pleasant as possible. And think of the reward when you have gone through the treatment. When you have finally completed it and your worries are over.

Worry and guilt can be associated to lower premolars and upper molar teeth and to the stomach and pancreatic gland.

There he was, fighting for his life! He wanted to save him and do everything he could to keep him. He searched for other options, better solutions. But there was nothing else to do. It was definitely too late.

The heavy veil of sadness started to cover him. He should have taken care of him earlier. While there was still time.

They had exhausted their options. They could do nothing to save him. He had waited too long. All they could do was extract him. Tears ran down his cheeks and he felt the regret and the remorse of losing one of his closest allies. He was devastated. *Would the girls ever look at him again?*

He regretted his stubbornness. The late nights, the binge drinking, and the chain smoking.

One last look. One last glimpse. One last yearning. Gone. Gone forever. Now it is definite. He lost this tooth.

There it was. Staring back at him. The ugly, gaping hole. Where it had once lived.

Out of the corner of his eye he saw his dentist dropping it into the surgical bin. That was the end of his tooth.

After grasping the gravity of the situation, he swore to himself, *This will not happen to me again. From this point on I will definitely have my regular check-ups.*

All the should haves, could haves, did not dos, bring people to the situation they are facing now. They might be overwhelmed by sadness because they haven't taken the dental health steps they should have taken years ago when the situation was not that dire.

And now, they regret not listening to the advice of friends who encouraged them to look after their teeth.

Is it too late now? It does not always have to be. They might not achieve the results they could have obtained a few years back, however, it is very rare to have no hope. With new techniques and materials there are often options even if their dental situation is a very challenging one.

It is as it is.

Once they move from the passenger seat into the driver's seat there is no place and no time for shame, sadness or regret.

There is only moving forward.

Sadness and regret can be associated to lower molars and upper premolar teeth and to the large intestine and lungs.

4. Stress: The Chair

Her heart was beating fast. Her breathing faltering. Sweat on her forehead. There it was again. The same noise. Over and over again. A frightening noise. Then a scream from the room next door. She's on her own. Adrenaline pumping through her veins. Her heart pulsating in her ears. Panic!

The door opens slowly. There he is. She can see his silhouette. She is just about to freak out. Should she run or stay? Then she hears his voice. A very deep voice.

"Hello Dorothy, please take a seat." Her dentist guides her to the chair.

She just about makes it to the chair. Her blood pressure increases, her heart rate speeds up, her breathing gets faster and her stress levels peak. Weak-kneed and terrified, she mumbles, "Just a check-up, please."

You have probably heard of people who are stressed just by the thought of sitting in the dentist chair. Any kind of action at the surgery can easily cause stress of different sorts for different people.

Maybe it is the anxiety lurking because you do not know what to expect once you sit down and open wide.

All the information from the internet about what can go wrong with dental treatments. You feel you're drowning in the overload of facts, figures and details. The online search did not really help to calm you down.

Maybe the voice in your head is playing mind games. What terrible things will happen, now that you have gathered enough courage to finally visit the dentist? You might even have experienced unpleasant painful procedures at a previous dentist. That's where your dental phobia stems from.

Ongoing levels of negative stress can create further dental problems like tooth grinding, tooth clenching and too much stress makes your body acidic. Acidity is the foundation for illnesses.

Stress also exhausts your adrenal glands and your thyroid which makes recovery from treatment more challenging.

With so much going on in your mouth and overall health you most likely do not know where to begin. You feel lost. Stressed out. Angry.

Wouldn't *now* be the best time to find an expert? An expert who really understands and can explain all these confusing and overwhelming findings. Someone who shows you the bigger picture concerning your health challenges and who can support you on your journey.

And together you create a simple step-by-step plan that moves you out of your health misery. Away from the stress and away from the anger. Towards resolution.

5. Anger and Rage: The Instructions

It just wouldn't work. No matter how hard he tried. It simply did not work! These bloody companies. *Why can't they write instructions everyone can understand?* He could feel the pressure rising in his throat.

Or was it him? Two left hands? Like his mum always said.

The pressure rose to irritation and then to frustration. His face reddened, his blood pressure culminating. His anger was about to explode into rage. Then something stopped him. A voice deep inside arose, *Stop the anger, Stop the rage. It is not getting you anywhere.* Surprised, he looked around. But there was no one there. It really did come from within him.

All of a sudden, he realized he had a choice. He could throw the parts across the room and break them or calm down, take a break and have a cup of tea, giving himself time to think. Those anger management classes really had worked wonders. He surprised himself.

Holding the package titled, *Become Your Own Dentist,* he realized it wasn't such a good idea to repair his own teeth after all.

Many believe it is other people or things that make them angry. Nothing could be further from the truth. This is a misperception. No person, no event, no external situation or incident has the magical power to make us angry. Feeling angry, like any other emotion, is a choice that we make.

Anger is often used to cover up other emotions such as fear, hurt, guilt or sadness. However, anger can also be used in a positive way. Anger can create change in your world inside and outside.

This motivation can either be used as a stick to get away from something undesired or as a carrot to move towards something desired. Depending on your choice, you can either focus on the problem or on the solution. It is a decision. Your decision.

Only when used in a destructive way will anger become a negative force. We can see it in a person's facial expression, their body language, their physiological responses and sometimes as pure aggression.

Unresolved anger whether conscious or unconscious, leads to resentment and bitterness and it can damage relationships, careers, health and teeth.

Anger and aggression can be associated with the canine teeth and to the liver and gall bladder.

6. FEAR: THE TRAP

Drops of cold sweat on his brow. His hands are damp. His feet are cold. His body is shaking. A frog in his throat. Nerves exposed. There is no going back now. No excuses. No plan B. It is happening. He cannot tell anybody about this. They would just laugh at him.

Is there a way out? A way to avoid this angst, dread, terror! Piling up in his mind. Filling his thoughts. One more minute. It is his time. Now!

One wish. Only one. To disappear off the face of the earth.

He hears his name. They have come for him. They wait. He must deliver. The stage is all his and he must perform.

Some people rate public speaking as their worst fear. But for others the fear of going to the dentist is even worse. There is so much to fear at the dentist. Feeling handcuffed in the chair. Completely and utterly at the dentist's mercy.

The electric stabbing pain that goes right into your face. The sharp needles you can feel penetrating your gum. The high-pitched sound piercing your ears. The stench of burnt tooth invading your nasal passages. The much-feared drill digging deeper and deeper into your tooth. The terrifying choking and gagging from too much water.

The extortionate costs ripping a massive hole in your budget. The treatment, possibly totally unnecessary treatment. The numbness giving your face a debilitated look. And the inability to say anything with your mouth wide open.

Making a fool out of yourself, panic attacks, the choking, the embarrassment, so many things that can go wrong, did go wrong. Just the thought of it makes the fear creep up faster than you wish for.

Allowing fear to run your life guarantees you won't succeed. Fear can freeze you. Can immobilise you. Not a very helpful state to be in if you want to resolve a problem. Fear of dental treatment has you focused on the one thing you want to avoid. How good are your chances of getting away from something if you constantly think of it?

A better way to deal with dental fear is to use its positive, motivational aspect and look for the reasons why the fear is there in the first place. Then remove the causes and get on with life.

Everything in your body is interconnected.

Nothing in us is wasted or useless.

Your oral health is directly related to your overall health and the other way around. Show me your teeth and I will tell you your story!

I have seen quite a few many patients who have suffered from diseases in their urogenital system, treated the infected tooth and got rid of the problem.

Fear is the emotion correlated with your upper and lower front teeth, kidneys, bladder and urogenital system.

7. Denial: The Mirror

"Denial ain't just a river in Egypt." Mark Twain's words echoed in her mind. She is upset. Her dentist was clear about it, she caught her out. But she does not want to accept the facts. The facts have been there for a long time. The evidence built up over many years. But she would rather reject it instead, sweeping it all under the carpet. Insisting it cannot be true. *It happens to other people, not me.* Despite the overwhelming evidence, it was crystal clear. She did not want to face it. So, she ignored it.

She had suffered for years. In silence. In pain. Telling no one. Not even her closest friends. She was too embarrassed and far too frightened. What would they think? She found excuse after excuse. They believed her.

Not this time. Not with the new dentist. This time she was made to face reality. She confronted her with the truth. Made her look into the mirror. Made her look closely into her mouth. The fear overtook her entire body and she could deny it no longer. Reality was staring back at her. Her teeth were terribly wobbly, decayed and her gums massively infected.

In ostrich-like-fashion you can bury your head in the sand and pretend you are ok, knowing full well you are not. But how does denial help with your dental problems? It is the fear of what could happen that you do not want to face. This drives you into denial. And denial disempowers you.

There are things going on in your mouth that you do not want to know about. Things, that if you knew about, you would be doing something about, and you would take action.

The fact is that you are denying yourself the knowledge that damage is happening to you, that you are not taking this into consideration and *you* are allowing this to happen.

Denial finds great excuses with phrases like, "I cannot do anything about it, because I do not have the time. I cannot afford it. It won't work for me." Only more reasons for you not to take action.

Denial prolongs the time until you finally have to face the fact that you cannot leave it any longer. All the time this damage is worsening in your mouth. This damaging behaviour is affecting your entire body in so many different ways and you are not controlling it. You are not dealing with it, although it is literally killing you.

So, overcome your fear. Stop denying yourself. Your health. Take responsibility and do something about it. Now.

Even if your budget is limited you can start your journey by getting an overview of your current situation. Then, together with a dentist, who looks at you as a whole rather than just at your teeth, come up with a plan that prioritises the most urgent problems and gets you going.

This way, you know what needs to be done and you can create a step-by-step plan to achieve your goal of the best oral health you can imagine.

If you do not get going you will blame yourself later.

How could he? How could my parents not have stopped him? How could they be so ignorant? How dare he take my teeth out?

She remembers the traumatic extractions very well. She was only twelve years old. She never forgave them. Not her parents. Nor the dentist.

They said it was to make space for the other teeth. And he took out four perfectly healthy teeth. Pre-emptively! Because my mouth was too small. Ha! What a joke! That's not what my friends said!

And now. Fifteen years later, look what's happened. The wisdom teeth are still impacted. My teeth then had so much freedom they gravitated West and now I have a wonky smile.

Could he not do something else? Was there not another option? Something that would have really helped. Why did my parents insist on this? Force me to have it done. They are to blame.

It is unbelievable. I should file a complaint about him. I. Am. Furious!

Blame and resentment are two of those emotions that can easily be triggered by life events. But what happens if we blame or resent others?

It is often easier to blame and resent others rather than accept the part that we played in the situation. But aren't blame and resentment just excuses that supposedly keep us safe? That protect us in our comfort zone without the need to directly take responsibility for our position? Isn't it easier to put the onus onto someone else?

However, it comes with a price.

Think about it for a moment. How do blame and resentment really help you? What has happened cannot be undone. By blaming and resenting yourself or others you give your power away.

Is there a secret satisfaction, a secondary gain, that we obtain by making somebody else wrong and ourselves right? Ultimately, this leads you to become the victim or the martyr, damaging your own well-being with the inability to take responsibility for your actions.

Everything you have achieved in your life as well as the things you haven't achieved are a direct manifestation of how you treat yourself and others. It is not how someone else has treated you.

The most important lessons here are to take responsibility and become accountable for your own feelings. To move beyond the blame and the resentment. To get to a point where you are healed, where you release these emotions, where you forgive and where you learn to love.

Otherwise more dis-ease will be created.

The wisdom teeth are the teeth often involved with these emotions and they are linked to the small intestine and heart.

9. SHAME: THE RECKONING

She looks into the mirror. What a mess, she still can't believe it.

Why didn't I do something? Anything, when it all started, before it got so bad?

Every time she looks in the mirror and sees those rotten teeth and bleeding gums staring back at her, she feels more and more embarrassed. Totally ashamed. Those brown, decayed and wobbly teeth are the worst teeth she's ever seen. They look disgusting. She feels the tears welling in her eyes. Here comes the overwhelm. "NOOOOooooooo!"

How could she be so stupid? Why did she leave it so long? And worse still, her face looks fifteen years older than she actually is. Her breath stinks—no wonder no one wants to come close. When was the last time she kissed someone? No wonder she can't get a man.

And worse than that, she has to pay yet another bill to get the mess sorted.

Indignant, she glares at herself! It is not just her teeth and gums that have suffered. She feels the effect in her stomach too. She can't chew properly, which her stomach doesn't appreciate. She is constipated and bad tempered. The list goes on.

She is terrified about the lecture she'll get from her dentist. Accused of wilful neglect, she is ashamed by her own lack of awareness.

Nowadays is there any excuse for missing or rotten teeth?

Absolutely! The reason being, emotions play a massive part in preventing you from seeing your dentist on a regular basis. If you are ashamed by the state of your teeth and the fact that you haven't visited your dentist, then you are not alone.

And believe me, us dentists do understand.

Especially when front teeth are involved, where everyone can easily spot it at first sight. Ugly or missing teeth can make a person feel truly ashamed.

Interestingly, most dentists are actually very empathetic when their patients feel embarrassed. From a dentist's perspective the situation looks different all together. They have seen it all before and they have been trained to support you and to care for you.

It is likely you have noticed people who hold their hand over their mouth when speaking. They do not want you to see what is missing, or perhaps, what you would see is not very inviting to look at, or they suffer from bad breath. These are all reasons they may feel ashamed. Some people might even stop talking, smiling or laughing all together out of shame that someone may discover the bad state of their teeth.

Do not let shame prevent you from getting the help you need. Shame can go as far as preventing people leaving their homes. They do not want to go out anymore. They do not want to run the risk of having to show their face, their teeth.

This can contribute to social isolation, feeling outlawed, excluded. It can even lead to depression.

The teeth primarily involved with shame are the lower second molars linked with the stomach and pancreas.

10. DEPRESSION: THE TURNAROUND

Christine was a happy, healthy young girl of thirteen when the dentist had to do the first filling on her first lower left molar. He didn't have to drill much. But he filled it with this dark, grey, silver filling. Mercury amalgam.

A few months later the pain crept in, pain all over her body. Her memory started to decline. It became so bad she couldn't even concentrate properly in school. Her previously excellent marks were turned upside down. She was in tears a lot of the time for no apparent reason. Hardly recognisable, she was a shadow of her former self.

Her digestion was impaired, she had put on weight. A lot of weight! She could see herself getting bigger and bigger. As a young girl this is not what you want to see when you look in the mirror.

She became anxious, fearful, distressed. She refused to go out anymore or meet with friends. Her self-esteem plummeted. She felt very, very depressed. A feeling unknown to her before. She even had thoughts of suicide.

None of the medical tests shed any light on this grave matter. She was put onto numerous medications by the doctors, almost like a guinea pig: antibiotics, steroids, anti-depressants. Nothing made any difference.

The GP and her headmaster couldn't make any sense out of her symptoms and believed she was making it up to get attention. They decided to section her. For her own safety. To give her time to think about her apparently dishonest behaviour.

Three days before her sectioning, Christine and her mum came into my practice in tears. They told me their story and upon examination I discovered the tiny mercury amalgam filling that had contributed to mercury poisoning.

I agreed to talk to the GP and headmaster in a bid to obtain a six-week period of grace whereby we could commence treatment, to which they agreed.

Removing this one tiny mercury amalgam filling together with a profound detoxification programme, saved her life. This saved her from going mad, from being sectioned and freed her from medication and got her back to a happy and healthy life within two months.

Depression and anxiety go hand in hand. Depression can affect anyone. Poor dental health can trigger feeling depressed.

Depression is sometimes seen as unexpressed anger turning inwards, consuming the sufferer from the inside. Therefore, it is important to deal with depression as soon as it becomes obvious.

Depression can come from emotional pain like the traumatic loss of a friend, a pet or a tooth. Depression has ruined lives. It even contributes to people choosing to end their lives.

It can also be triggered entirely by environmental causes such as heavy metals, pesticides, herbicides, formaldehyde, solvents or food additives including monosodium glutamate (MSG), artificial sweeteners such as aspartame, sulphites used as preservatives in food, the Epstein-Barr virus or even an electrolyte deficiency.

For many years, there has been a rumour that dentists, above all other professions, have the highest rate of depression and suicide. One may wonder if those affected are the ones who are still using mercury amalgam fillings.

Antidepressant drugs can cause dry mouth which can support the development of tooth decay, gum disease and bad breath. And it lowers blood pressure.

Many patients heal from depression by having their mercury amalgam fillings replaced with less toxic materials or by changing their diet: refraining from wheat, dairy, sugar and artificial additives such as MSG. Research shows that switching to a mainly organic diet with lots of vegetables can contribute to this result.

Depression is definitely not something you have to live with.

The teeth linked to depression are the upper premolars and the lower first and second molars. The organs that relate to these teeth are the lungs and large intestine, both have to do with letting go.

11. ACCEPTANCE AND GRATITUDE: THE SPOT

He had been concerned about this dark black spot for a long time. It was on his mind a lot. Actually, it was on the end of his nose, but he still worried about it. A lot. He should do something about it but he feared the diagnosis. It just didn't look right. There was something sinister about it.

Thinking too much about it and what it could be, brought him to the brink of feeling almost depressed. He did not like that feeling. Nor did he like the spot.

Then, he looked at it again. What he saw was not to his liking. The small dark spot had grown even bigger. For weeks it was level with the skin but now it was above skin level. And it was itchy.

His close friends made him face reality. "It's not normal" they said, "Get it looked at!"

With all the courage he could muster, he rang the surgery and got an appointment. The days until the doctor could see him were a constant rollercoaster of feelings. Fear, denial. *It cannot be that bad, can it?* Then worry and depression.

He was really grateful when the day of the appointment arrived and he would know once and for all what was going on. When the doctor said, "Early stage of skin cancer," he was not really surprised. It was what his fear was about. To hear the C word.

Now that he had heard it, he felt a mixture of terror and relief. Now that he knew what it was, could he deal with the truth of it? He remembered a friend who had recovered from skin cancer and had once told him that the first thing he had done was to accept the situation. Though it was hard to do, he must accept it for what it was.

There was nothing to debate about. It is what it is. Accepting what is, is the start of the healing.

Somehow, he just wondered how he had attracted this. *Why is this happening to me?*

Remembering what his friend had said, he could not be scared into rushing a decision to receive any kind of mainstream cancer therapy. Instead he would pay a visit to his friend who does all kind of weird stuff. His friend had somehow miraculously healed himself from skin cancer. So, if he could do it, he was sure he could too.

Whether it's a decayed tooth, a gum infection or any other illness, as soon as you accept the truth of your present state and deal with your feelings about it, your situation will shift just by having changed your perspective and healing can start.

A wave of gratitude came over him. Gratitude to know he was not on his own. Gratitude to know that there was a solution. Gratitude that he could conquer his fears and that he had taken the first step; facing this challenge and moving towards his recovery.

With the support of his friend he cleared himself without any drugs or surgery. Four months later nothing was left of the dark brown spot. Conventional medicine had no explanation for this miraculous healing.

Acceptance means embracing what is, rather than wishing for what is not.

If you find yourself in a challenging situation, acceptance might not be the first thing that springs to mind. And it might not be what you want to do. However, acceptance is more than just an emotion, it is also an attitude.

It can be tough to change one's state of mind. However, the rewards and benefits far outweigh the amount of effort invested in exploring and eventually overcoming limitations. The process of self-exploration is extremely rewarding and can indeed be transformative.

Gratitude is one of the most important personality traits. Gratitude is a feeling of appreciation and acceptance. Once you adopt a grateful attitude, you are more likely to experience situations you can be grateful for.

Gratitude makes us feel much better and it buffers against disempowering emotions. Both emotions, acceptance and gratitude, are an integral part of a healthy healing process.

The teeth related to gratitude and acceptance are the upper and lower front teeth linked with the kidneys and bladder.

12. WELL-BEING: THE DESTINATION

We all want to be well. However, well-being is much more than the absence of illness. Well-being is what we strive for. Well-being is about balancing our thoughts, beliefs, values, feelings and behaviour to support us in our day-to-day lives.

A positive outlook is a fundamental aspect of living a happy, healthy and well-balanced life.

Well-being can be summarised as how we feel about ourselves and our life.

Our mental and emotional well-being can be threatened on a daily basis with things such as dental and medical problems, financial stress, family issues or relationship challenges, to name just a few.

Once all dental and medical issues have been addressed, we can move towards maintaining equanimity.

With well-being comes love. Love for yourself. Love for others. Love for the things you do.

Once you start to take responsibility for your own health, you can be proud of the fact that you did. You have moved away from those negative emotions and limiting beliefs, towards a healthy mindset on all levels: physical, emotional, mental and spiritual.

Well-being is strongly linked with joy, happiness and life satisfaction. And, of course with love for oneself and peace of mind. You know it when you have it. When you are there, pat yourself on the back for going on the journey, facing your demons and conquering them.

If you have experienced challenges in life and have overcome them, now you too can be an inspiration to others and a role model to guide and motivate them. Let them be part of your journey and guide them on their own way. Out of their misery. The way you walked out of yours.

LIFESTYLE
RUNNING YOUR BODY

We have established how emotions can affect the body and the important role they play in your health. Now you will discover how your lifestyle choices affect your oral and overall health and how to decide upon the best options for you.

"A routine treatment," they told him. Normally. However, this time it had gone horribly wrong. He became increasingly concerned, mouth wide open, staring at the hypnotic poster on the ceiling, as the dentist whispered, "Damn!"

He moved his gaze and saw the panic in his dentist's frightened eyes. The sheer horror of disbelief. "Do not move, do not move!" the dentist commanded. Then he felt it. The sting at the back of the throat, the blockage in his airways.

"I can't bweeve, I can't bweeve," he gasped, choking. *Get that damned thing out of my throat,* he thought. *Now! It cannot end like this. I don't want to die!*

In one final, desperate move the terrified dentist managed to grab the end of the root canal needle and catapulted it into the tray just in the nick of time, before his patient expired.

Two lives saved. Two bodies soaked in sweat. Two hearts pounding like mad. One saved from a near fatal incident, the other saved from a painful lawsuit.

Although we know that we would die without oxygen, no one teaches us how to breathe correctly and this is something we definitely do not learn at school or as babies. Proper breathing is using your diaphragmatic muscle. That is why it is also called diaphragmatic breathing, deep breathing or belly breathing.

If you cannot breathe properly, you cannot think properly.

When you breathe deeply, the air comes in through your nose fully, fills your lungs, and your lower belly rises. You feel the expansion low down in your lungs.

Diaphragmatic breathing brings with it many benefits such as:

- reduced anxiety,
- improved blood flow,
- increased energy levels,
- improved posture,

Diaphragmatic breathing stimulates the lymphatic system, helping to detox the body and acting as a natural painkiller.

Mums can actually help their newborn babies to breathe correctly by breastfeeding them. Breastfeeding helps to develop the baby's breathing pathways as well as their jawbones and places their teeth and tongue in the correct position.

Diaphragmatic breathing improves your body chemistry by bringing sufficient oxygen into your lungs and exhaling toxic carbon dioxide. Shallow breathing doesn't do that.

Shallow breathing, or breathing through your mouth, can lead to all sorts of diseases such as allergies, asthma, problems with the tonsils, middle ear infections, poor dental conditions, sleeping disorders, snoring and sleep apnoea.

Sleeping disorders are a very serious problem, reducing the oxygen supply which can affect the regeneration that normally occurs during sleep.

The good news is: proper breathing can be learned. And deep breathing is a fantastic stress release.

You cannot blame your genetics for not breathing properly.

2. Hydration

He starts digging straight after breakfast. Two cups of black coffee, his usual breakfast. Coffee keeps him going, gives him energy.

Garden work. He loves his garden. There is always something to do and he hardly ever takes a break. Digging holes for trees, breaking up the soil to plant new seeds, pruning and weeding. Even if it is boiling hot like it is today.

He didn't pay attention to his thirst until he feels the parched dryness hitting the back of his throat like a piece of sandpaper on dried wood. A horrible feeling. All of a sudden, he thinks of nothing else except water. His body takes over. He must drink. The body dehydrated, desperate for moisture.

Suddenly, his muscles tighten. The agonizing cramp starts to creep up his legs. A skull-bursting shooting pain hit him like a bolt out of the blue. His whole body spins in anguish.

Thirst! A burning thirst. His tongue glued to his gums, so dry and sticky. He needs water, now. Dizziness blurs his vision.

Like a mirage in the distance his water source, the shed, seems so far away. *Must reach the water, must reach the shed!*

On all fours he crawls desperately to the shed. Inch by inch. He is so disoriented, he doesn't even know he has made it until he bangs his head on the shed door. He pushes it with all his might, crawling into the dark, cool space and reaches out in desperation.

His hand finds the bottle and just in time.

His body starts to shake. He can barely get the bottle to his mouth quickly enough. Close to exhaustion, he manages to take a big gulp and feels the relief of the cool liquid running down his throat. Euphoria hits him, his body rejoices. He feels the life slowly coming back into him.

Depending on your age, up to 75% of your body is water. The brain consists of up to 90% water. Water, like air, is essential for life.

We need water for almost all the processes in our body and we need a lot of it. You should provide your body with at least 1.5 litres of clean water daily, depending upon your activity level.

Lack of water is the source of many diseases as well as pain. A deficiency of only 2% water will lead to severe physical and intellectual restrictions.

Clean and pure water is hardly ever what you get when turning on the tap or from plastic bottles.

Water is far more than just a thirst quencher.

Only when you drink pure, clean water will your body be able to utilise it optimally for its internal cleansing processes. Contaminated water has to be cleaned first by the body which rids it of energy and leaves only a little water for the purposes it was meant for.

Drinking water from a clean well, a trustworthy source, placed in glass bottles or using a really good water filtration system, is as important as putting the right fuel into your car's engine.

Fruit and vegetables supply the body with very good water infused with electrolytes. However, alcohol, coffee, fizzy drinks and black tea strip the body of water. Drinking coffee, black tea or alcohol dehydrates your body.

If you feel thirsty, your body has already been dehydrated for much longer than you realise.

Often people think they are hungry, but in fact their body is craving water not food.

If you think malnutrition is a Third World problem, think again!

Despite oversized portions, the Western world is starving. We are starved of nutrient-rich foods.

People are constantly hungry, always eating, non-stop snacking and craving for something. Much of the time their craving is simply an emptiness which they wish to fill. Food fills that emptiness. And they are eating the wrong food. They starve themselves whilst consuming overfilled plates. Do you find this hard to believe?

More and more adults, and even children, are suffering from obesity: simply because the food they eat is not really food at all. It is a combination of chemical additives and dehydrated toxic fats, fillers mixed with flavour enhancers made to look like food.

No matter how much food they put in their mouths, it is not calming their hunger because the body needs something that it is simply not getting. The body can only operate efficiently when it is given the correct nutrients. It craves these.

There is a disease epidemic because bodies are not getting the necessary foods. People are slowly killing themselves by feeding their bodies food that lacks nutrients.

The first symptoms may appear in the forms of weight gain, bleeding gums, tooth decay, loss of energy and depression, to name a few.

Living on junk food not only makes you fat, it also makes you sick. We are what we eat. It is that simple. Unfortunately, we are no longer eating according to our nature.

For your body to operate like a finely-tuned, high-performance engine, consuming processed food stuffed with sugar and artificial sweeteners will not deliver.

Although there is no one-size-fits-all diet, there are, however, some fundamental rules which apply to everyone. Talk to your health practitioner or nutritionist to discover the diet that suits you best.

Eat food the way nature delivers it. Raw, uncooked and unrefined. Reduce your sugar intake, keep coffee and alcohol consumption to a minimum. Steer clear of genetically modified grains including corn, soy and wheat, monosodium-glutamate, farmed fish, hydrogenated fats and everything artificial, especially sweeteners. And reduce dairy as much as possible

Dr Weston Price, the famous American dentist, discovered through his travels to remote tribes that their simple diet did not allow for tooth decay, gum disease or any kind of chronic degenerative diseases to develop.

Drinking pasteurised and homogenised cow's milk, to prevent osteoporosis, is just one bogus story we still get told. Even as it is skyrocketing in countries where people gulp milk by the gallon.

If you want to take advantage of the benefits of milk, you have to drink it raw, untreated, or as kefir. Raw milk is high in vitamin D and iodine. Pasteurisation kills most of the enzymes and good bacteria, denatures most of the amino acids and proteins, damages most of the vitamins and minerals and makes the calcium basically unusable for your body. Homogenisation of milk is even worse as it turns the previously good fats into toxic fats.

Better still, to get the correct form of calcium into your body eat lots of green vegetables (such as broccoli, kale, brussels sprouts) or sardines, white beans and figs.

The number of people suffering from chronic diseases is increasing, with little hope for a cure from mainstream medicine. Observing what we feed ourselves can answer many questions.

A well-balanced diet cannot avert extreme disasters or severe emotional events, but it is essential for any subsequent healing process and contributes towards the prevention of chronic disease.

4. SUPPLEMENTATION

She had been complaining of chronic tiredness and lack of energy for years. Her family had finally had enough. In one last, desperate attempt to get to the bottom of her ill health she consulted a holistic dentist, recommended by a friend.

It was first discovered on an X-ray. A deep, dark and dangerous-looking bone infection. The operation was scheduled. She arrived on time. She was even allowed to have breakfast. No general anaesthetic required. All preparations made.

The procedure started. The dentist was optimistic. However, he underestimated the scale of the infection. Masses of soft, infected bone. Disgusting oily, brownish liquid seeped out of the bone. A vile smell followed. He thoroughly scraped the bone until no soft tissue remained. He even used ozone to kill the bacteria. What was left was a massive hole in the bone. He filled it with plasma from her own blood, placed the stitches. Job done. The surgery went well. Another satisfied customer. Or so he thought.

The complications started two days later. Pulsating pain in the bone. Foul taste in her mouth. Swollen gums. Along with a high temperature came the shaking and the feeling of nausea. The surgery area looked empty. Dry socket is what they call it. And it is excruciatingly painful.

A second surgery was needed. The same procedure. Clean-fill-stitch. This time it will heal, the dentist assured her. No. It did not. More pain, more nausea. She could not eat any food and had to live on pain killers.

Her blood tests showed very low levels of vitamin D, vitamin C, magnesium, zinc, iron and other minerals and vitamins. All essential for proper bone and tissue healing. She was asked to supplement these nutrients over the next few days. Still the pain remained. She had to go for further surgery which included high-dose intravenous vitamin C.

Third time lucky. Same procedure. This time she healed.

Some experts still claim that supplementation is just a rip-off to part you from your hard-earned cash. These are often the same ones who state that you still get all your nutritional requirements from grains, dairy, fruits, meat and vegetables.

For many years my experience has been very different.

Supplementation nowadays is a vital requirement. This is mainly due to modern farming methods which create a quick turnaround of crops, resulting in the depletion of vital minerals in the soil. Our fruits and vegetables, even the organically grown ones, lack minerals and vitamins and so do we when we eat them.

Minerals are the spark plugs of life. If we do not get enough of them, our body cannot function optimally. The same is true for vitamins. Some can be produced by our body, whereas others have to be supplemented with our diet.

This becomes very evident in dentistry where bleeding gums, tooth decay and receding bone levels are on the increase and we see diet-related chronic illnesses like diabetes or Crohn's disease skyrocketing.

Especially when undergoing dental surgery, it is recommended that you support the healing process pre- and post-surgery with a specially designed supplementation protocol.

However, it must be remembered that supplements are not a substitute for a well-balanced healthy diet and food-based natural supplements are more beneficial than those which are synthetically produced.

5. Gut Health

It started with a simple flu that lingered and refused to leave. Stronger medicine was required. That's how the attack started. With antibiotics.

The strike came without warning. For all of them it was a hostile attack. Only the very lucky ones survived. A terrible assault from their host. Most of them died instantly. The good and the bad ones. Killed by the flood of toxins. Killed by the antibiotics. The bugs had no time to mourn.

They would quickly analyse their nemesis because they knew the next onslaught was literally only hours away. They knew it. Their ancestors had been there before, they had been warned. They were lacking reinforcements. Antibodies must be produced to give them immunity. Their defences must be strengthened.

Gone are the good times. They had to work together and fast. They knew "What doesn't kill us makes us stronger." Future generations depended upon it. This would create a better future. A much brighter future.

One day these antibiotic attacks would be nothing more than a walk in the park for those immune little bugs. Welcomed, to charge their batteries, give them something to get their teeth into. This would flex their muscles and get them ready for the next war. And slowly, but steadily would lead to the takeover of the entire human body.

No antibiotic would ever harm them again. They will be immune.

They will be the *Super-Bad-Bugs*! Ready, for world domination.

Health and fitness magazines are full of them. Skinny models with barely a layer of epidermis on their bones. Many of them do not look healthy, but the wonders of Photoshop make them so.

In our Western World being overweight or gaining weight, especially around the hips, is not the ideal body type most people aspire to. However, there are many different body shapes. And where you are putting weight on shows what is happening within your body.

Men who tend to get man boobs have quite a low testosterone level. Stress-eating creates a more apple-shaped body because the fat accumulates higher up.

It appears that a pear-shaped body indicates unhealthy lifestyle, incorrect diet and suggests the bearer's gut health is far from optimal. A pear-shaped body is also a sign of hormonal imbalance and toxins amassing around the hips.

Bad nutrition = Bad gut health

Being overweight decreases your life expectancy and increases the risk for all sorts of chronic diseases such as diabetes or heart disease. A healthy gut flora is what we want to provide our bodies with.

A properly functioning and digesting gut is the absolute cornerstone of your overall health. Without a healthy gut it is impossible to stay or become healthy, because a large part of your immune system is located in the gut. Antibiotics destroy your gut bacteria. Soon, humans will no longer be able to control any infection at all. With the gut flora dead, we are susceptible to all sorts of chronic diseases and are likely to be killed by our own hands.

Digestion starts the moment you bring food into your mouth. No, in fact, it actually starts the moment you think of the food you are going to eat. As soon as your brain receives the information, *food arriving to be digested*, it starts an entire cascade of programmes that produce hormones, saliva and enzymes, beginning the digestive process.

Therefore, it is important to chew properly and masticate the food into the smallest possible pieces. Swallowing down big chunks of food overburdens your stomach. It is also best to eat when you are relaxed, away from the TV or any mobile phones. Being mindful when eating actually improves digestion.

To support your gut in doing its job properly, it is important that you allow it to rest in- between meals. This you can easily do by intermittent fasting. Intermittent fasting is achieved by having your last meal around 6pm then not eating until midday the next day. Intermittent fasting supports your body's daily three eight-hour cycles of elimination, digestion and absorption.

Between the hours of 4am and 12pm your body is eliminating. This is the cycle most important for cleansing and releasing toxins.

Between the hours of 12pm and 8pm your body is digesting. This is the cycle most important for digesting, metabolising and burning your food. Therefore, this is the period when meals should be eaten. Furthermore, only eat when you are hungry. Eat small and colourful portions from small plates.

Between the hours of 8pm and 4am your body is absorbing. This is the cycle most important for absorbing nutrients and transporting them to your cells. This is also the time when healing, regeneration and renewing of cells takes place.

Adhering to this natural rhythm makes it easier to digest food properly, prevents you from weight fluctuation and keeps you more alert. Try this for four weeks and notice the changes yourself.

The simplest and cheapest way to determine if your gut is healthy and your digestion works properly, is a very easy test. Just ask yourself, "How much toilet paper do I need?"

The amount of toilet paper you need to clean up is a great indicator. If your digestion works well, you will only need little to no paper!

6. Sunlight

The scene is set. Just like a movie. The plane lands on the airstrip in the midday sun. Mavis and Archie have arrived in Benidorm for their dream holiday. They haven't had one in years.

As the cabin door opens, Mavis is the first one out. "It's bleeding hot out here," she shrieks back at Archie, who is in tow. "Oh good, just how I like it," he replies.

Having left the airport and after the twelfth stop, the coach finally arrives at their hotel and they're off. Checked in—bags thrown into their hotel room, swimsuit on—and that's just Archie. Mavis comes rushing after him in her two-piece and together they make their way down to the crowded pool to enjoy their first afternoon of cocktails and sunshine on their all-inclusive package holiday.

It's 2pm and they are already on their third cocktail, plastered *and* plastered in sunscreen. Four hours later, they wake up, slightly tipsy and roasted.

They make their way back to their room and get ready for dinner. Having barely seen the sun in years, they both now have heat stroke and the cheap sunscreen has proved worse than useless. During dinner, skin red-raw, they are dehydrated and starting to feel ill. Archie cracks a joke, that Mavis is the same colour as the lobster he's eating.

Mavis gets the last laugh and so does the lobster as Archie is now complaining of toothache after cracking his tooth on his seafood platter! A fine start to a perfect holiday!

The experts have warned us that long exposure to the sun is dangerous to our health whilst the rates of skin cancer have skyrocketed in recent years.

However, using sunshine wisely has far greater health benefits than some scaremongering skin-cancer experts make us believe. What could be better than waking up to blue skies and sunshine, going outside and walking barefoot on dew-laden grass, feeling the sun's warming rays as they caress your skin with each step you take? Soaking the energy up into your body, you cannot help but feel uplifted, like the world is your oyster. These are the feelings we can get when we go on holiday.

Forgotten are all the fears and worries, the stresses and anxieties and all the other negativities of life. They all take a back seat to the good feeling that sunshine brings into our lives. Sunshine makes us feel happy and motivated.

How likely is it that you make better decisions when you have a more positive attitude? You might even feel brave enough to go to the dentist! Making this the first step to improving your dental health.

Sunlight has many different health benefits, amongst them pain reduction, a boost of feel-good hormones, reduced inflammation, the improvement of skin conditions and a lowering of high blood pressure.

For dental health, sunshine is important because it helps the body produce vitamin D, which is important for healthy teeth, gums, bones and for healing after any kind of surgery.

Without enough vitamin D we do not heal well, our teeth are more likely to decay and the bones become brittle, which can lead to osteoporosis.

About 75% of people in the Northern hemisphere are estimated to be vitamin D deficient. Avoiding sunshine is as risky as smoking.

Choose your sunscreen wisely because many have toxic ingredients, and be aware that sunscreen actually prevents the production of vitamin D.

7. Physical Activity

Yesterday evening his beloved dog, Tilla, his best friend of twelve years, had to be put to sleep. Devastated, he felt very guilty taking the decision to end his pet's life.

Today started as badly as the previous day had ended when he tripped over his shoes and hit his head on the door frame. Great! He now had a bleeding, painful cut on his forehead to exacerbate his misery. Then his computer had a meltdown, as did he when the IT guy did not answer the phone. With his frustration accelerating rapidly into rage he was just about to throw his laptop through the open window when something stopped him.

He grabbed his sports bag, his car keys and his jacket, slammed the front door behind him and drove to the gym to try to work off some of his frustration.

Still in a foul mood he started his warm-ups and shortly, as the endorphins started to kick in, he could feel his mood improving. He knew he had done the right thing by coming to the gym to do a workout. He blew off steam, became focused and moved his aggression into the weights and abreacted to the punch ball.

With the release of endorphins flooding his body, his neurochemistry changed and his mood dramatically improved.

After the session, whilst showering, he could feel how the physical exertion had improved his whole state of being, as he knew his body benefitted from regular exercise.

Physical activity changes your mood and puts you in a much happier frame. If you add to this some sunshine and deliciously nurturing food, you feel like you are on top of the world. This is the state you want to be in when making decisions. Like the decision to go to the dentist for a check-up!

When you feel good about yourself, about your life and your world, you are in a better mood to make better decisions.

It probably comes as no surprise that regular physical activity is an important part of a healthy lifestyle. The benefits you receive from performing any kind of regular exercise are tremendous.

Just a brisk walk will do a lot for your fitness. There is no real need for hour-long exercises, just ten minutes every other day will make a difference to the way you feel and will create quite an impact on your health.

You could also choose high-intensity interval training (HIIT) which transforms your health and endurance at an even higher level. Even walking up and down the stairs for a few minutes until you are out of breath, then stopping for thirty seconds before recommencing the exercise and repeating again will make a noticeable difference.

Regular exercise also has an impact on your oral health. It can prevent gum disease. Research also found that regular exercise goes hand in hand with reduced tooth decay. Obviously, you have to stay away from any kind of sports drinks. They are loaded with sugar and are far too acidic.

When you exercise you breathe more deeply. Deep breathing brings more oxygen into your lungs and your cells and you exhale more carbon dioxide. You activate your lymphatic system which helps clean your blood. And as a side effect, you produce a lot of feel-good hormones which help deal with your stress levels and balance your emotions.

Being in a better mood does not necessarily solve all your problems. But it definitely puts you in a better frame of mind where you can tap more fully into your available resources.

8. Sleep

The big meeting is tomorrow. She must be in top form. Going to bed early and getting a good night's sleep is vital.

He was tired and went to bed at the same time. She turns off the light, closes her eyes, gets very comfortable and… then it starts.

In her gentle slumber it sounds like distant thunder. The storm seems to get closer and before long is upon her. *OMG, she thinks, he's snoring again!*

She can't afford another sleepless night. She knows how detrimental a disturbed night is to her health, her sanity. She hates it when he snores. It is loud, it is deafening and it is unhealthy. She's tried ear plugs but they either pop out or they seem to absorb the sound to an even greater degree.

She thinks of her meeting in the morning. She has no choice. In desperation she gives him an almighty prod in his thigh. A wonderful silence fills the bedroom. Now she can enjoy the relaxing sleep she deserves. The sleep she desperately needs. To feel re-vitalised and to ensure she can perform at her best. At last, she drifts off into deep, peaceful sleep.

Sleep is one of the most important aspects of our lives and because we spend so much time asleep, it is important to make the best out of it.

We need sleep for our body to regenerate. Our resting place should be comfortable and quiet. It should preferably be dark—to produce sufficient amounts of our sleep hormone, melatonin.

Ideally your bedroom should be free of EMF radiation from Wi-Fi, mobile phones (turn them off) and electro-smog.

For good oral health, good sleeping patterns are essential. This means you should breathe through your nose with your mouth closed.

If you breathe with an open mouth, saliva dries out and it loses its protective property for your teeth and may even result in developing tooth decay. What's more, you are more likely to snore with an open mouth and especially when you lie on your back.

Another sleeping pattern that can affect your teeth is grinding or clenching. This not only damages your teeth but also the surrounding muscles, gum, bone and your TMJ.

If you suffer from a lot of stress, your adrenal glands might be exhausted which can make it difficult for you to either fall asleep, sleep through the night or wake up refreshed even after long hours in bed.

9. Environmental Toxins

You blissfully walk around in your home, believing it is this wonderful secure place. This is your sanctuary.

But your home is a toxic place. It is poisoning you and your family on a daily basis.

Even as you sleep, you receive your fair share of electromagnetic radiation from Wi-Fi and the mobile phone you keep beside your bed and inhale one of the most toxic threats to your health if you have mould somewhere in your house, lurking behind your walls or under the carpet. Each sleeping breath inhales the toxins from the brominated flame and fire-retardant mattress, carpet and curtains in your bedroom.

The next morning you start your day with a glass of supposedly fresh tap water. Not only does it smell of chlorine, it also gives you your first shot of countless toxins such as chlorine, fluorine compounds, arsenic, radium, aluminium, copper, lead, mercury, cadmium barium, hormones, nitrates, pesticides and many more, with even more to follow during the day.

Next, you take a shower. The lovely smelling shower gel contains sodium laureth sulphate and many other questionable ingredients, all of which are being soaked up into your skin and probably end up in your bloodstream. Then, in order to prevent perspiration, you apply a deodorant. The aluminium from the deodorant finds its way into your lymphatic glands, blocking their drainage capacity.

Now you fry your free-range eggs in a non-stick pan which adds a sprinkling of nasty chemicals as they almost always contain a chemical called PFOA which, according to the *American Cancer Society* and the *Centers for Disease Control and Prevention,* can affect growth, development, the liver, fertility and even cancer.

Eating your organic porridge heated up in a microwave oven isn't healthy either. According to a Swiss study, microwave-heated food elevates cholesterol levels, decreases red blood cell levels, haemoglobin and leucocytes and clogs your blood.

Already in a hurry, you gulp down cheap over-the-counter supplements filled with more additives than active ingredients.

You haven't even left the house yet and you are already set up with an unimaginable cocktail of toxins ready for the day ahead. You are walking around as a hazardous waste container.

Then you start frying your brain with every mobile phone call you make. EMFs are everywhere.

You swallow hormone-disruptive chemicals that leak from the plastic bottles you drink from all day long. You inhale the polluted air drifting into your car. You sit like sardines in tube trains, having to cope with all the sneezes, coughs and what have yous from your fellow passengers. On your way to work you pop by the travel clinic to get your vaccination shots for your next exotic holiday and receive yet another blow to your immune system.

And the list goes on and on and on....

Unfortunately, most people would rather believe in reassuring lies than opt for the somewhat inconvenient truth.

Already in 2005, a study found 287 toxins in the blood of newborn babies, 180 of which are known carcinogens, 217 are toxic to the brain and 208 can cause birth defects.

Add to this the devastating effects of the lack of breastfeeding, contaminated water, polluted air, poisoned soil and processed foods and you can easily imagine the consequences this will have on our children's development and overall health.

In dentistry, we use some of the most toxic materials which are still allowed to be used on human beings. Mercury in amalgam fillings, hormone-disrupting components in composite fillings and fluorides.

Our oceans are full of plastic waste and contaminated by radiation from the Fukushima fallout. The pictures of fish dying from their guts full of plastic and with cancerous lesions all over their bodies are heartbreaking.

Herbicides and pesticides, used by farmers to increase their yield, have devastating effects on our health. They are possibly the most critical factor in contributing to the development of multiple chronic diseases such as obesity, allergies, colitis, Crohn's disease, Alzheimer's, depression and cancer.

According to a group of scientists assembled by the World Health Organization, glyphosate, the main ingredient of the pesticide *Roundup*™ is probably carcinogenic to humans.

It is time to reclaim our health! We must start reducing the amount of toxins we inhale, swallow, put on and in our body and the toxins we produce which harm ourselves, others and nature.

10. MEDICATION

Drugs can kill. One medication they said. To keep the symptoms in check. One pill, three years ago. They gave him a diagnosis, a label. Now he is on drugs for life. No cure!

Today, he is on four more different drugs. "To deal with the side effects," they explained. They damn well knew this was coming. He did not. He, of course, trusted them. The gods in their white coats. He believed everything they told him. He believed they knew best, after all they were the experts.

Nothing has helped. Now he is desperately searching for another way. A solution to his pain. Away from this debilitating life.

It is more than just the poisonous effect of the drugs that have caused his life to be such a burden. It is the compounding effect of all the other toxins from negative emotions, antibiotic resistant superbugs, nutritionally depleted food and the environmental toxins that have amplified his need for change.

"Are your teeth alright?" a friend asked. *A strange question,* he thought. He had no clue. So, he asked a holistic dentist to have a look at them. Surprisingly, everything the dentist said made perfect sense.

His root canaled teeth were removed, mercury fillings were replaced and the bone infections which he had no idea about were cleaned out thoroughly.

Within days he felt better. Now ten months later, no more symptoms, no more medication. Just the twitch in his big toe which reminds him of those four years of hell. He has finally got his life back!

No doubt, certain drugs have their place in medicine, or do they? However, taking a closer look cannot hurt.

Why do they call them *side effects*?

The only difference to the main effects is, that the side effects are not wished for. But that does not mean it is a side effect. Sooner or later you will need a different drug that counteracts the side effects of the drug which counteracted the first side effects.

50% of those over 65 in the UK take at least five different drugs.

If you check different medications, you will find that the named side effects in one medication is indeed the main reason for taking another drug.

Looking even more closely into clinical drug trials there is research to suggest that many of them are scientifically invalid and fraudulent from the offset.

Medical practitioners have to carefully assess which medication they can give to their patients. If a dentist uses adrenalin in an anaesthetic, it can cause problems with some patients. Some epileptic drugs can cause gum swelling and bleeding. Painkillers can cause stomach problems.

The challenge with most pharmaceutical drugs is that they are merely symptom suppressors rather than cause eliminators.

On a bigger scale, millions of unused pills are washed down the toilet together with the remains of the swallowed ones in urine and faeces, polluting our water supplies and ultimately the population with unwanted side effects.

11. No-Nos

Have you ever visited a friend in hospital or been there yourself? What did you think of the food they served? Was it tasty, fresh, full of raw ingredients, nutritious and healthy?

Most have experienced exactly the opposite. Bland, overcooked meals that contain lots of canned foods that need no proper chewing. Your teeth and your overall health will suffer massively from supervised neglect like this. Even if you survive the surgery and the super bugs, the food they offer could kill you. It is often light years away from being healthy and supportive to your healing process.

The place where you should be fed the very best and most nutritious food, to support the recovery process, immediately lets you down by dishing out cheap, tasteless and nutrient-free meals.

If you want a healthy body, are suffering or recovering from an illness here are a few foods to keep away from.

Sugar. Whether it is white sugar, artificial sweeteners or high fructose corn syrup. None of these have any nutritional value and are all poisons. Aspartame, for example, is linked to more than 100 detrimental health effects including mood swings, memory loss, chronic fatigue and diabetes.

Wheat. Wheat nowadays is totally different from how it was decades ago. The refined, bleached-white flour is essentially a sugar. It hardly has any nutritional value to it, just a bag full of very toxic chemicals from the production process.

Dairy. The problem starts by breeding cows who produce vast quantities of milk, feeding them soy-based food, enriched with antibiotics and hormones and other medication to keep them on their legs. Jammed in a cage where they can hardly move.

On top of this pasteurisation and homogenisation kill the milks enzymes. Without those enzymes milk becomes difficult to digest for humans. The same goes for cheese and yoghurt. Some say cow's milk is essentially for baby cows!

Other people advocate raw untreated milk from grass fed cows because it is still full of good stuff and is rich in iodine and vitamin D and its derivates such as full fat cheese or kefir.

Corn & Soy. They once were nutritious and healing, but GMO destroyed all that and nowadays there is only a very small percentage of unaltered crops remaining.

E-numbers. Check the labels for these ingredients and stay clear from artificial additives such as colourings or artificial flavourings or MSG.

Microwave ovens. Kills the food.

Meat. If meat is still part of your diet, buy only meat that is pasture-raised, grass-fed, free-range, organic and free of antibiotics. Stay away from pork, especially if you want to heal from a chronic disease.

Farmed Fish. Only opt for wild fish. Even those become more and more toxic. The higher in the food chain, the more toxic they are. Small fish = small toxicity!

Cook with Ghee or Coconut oil. Most other oils get damaged by high temperature. Use Olive oil for salads and other raw food.

Ancient physicians believed that healing was most effective when looking at the patient as a whole person as opposed to focusing on a specific illness, body part or symptom.

Being healthy is not simply the absence of an illness. It is a state of balance and harmony. Our ancient ancestors knew about the interconnection between mind, body and spirit and the environment within which we live. All are key factors to achieving homeostasis.

They also realized, long before the advent of antibiotics and X-rays, that a person's emotions and spirit played an important part in their healing process and staying healthy.

The ancient knowledge was kept sacred by the elders and shamans and passed on from generation to generation. Within their natural healing remedies, they also incorporated plant-based medicines, the origin of the herbal medicines and homeopathic remedies of today.

Modern orthodox medicine in the twentieth century brought with it some fantastic advancements in the treatment of acute injuries. However, the success of this approach is very limited when it comes to chronic disease as the symptom, rather than the cause, is treated.

The belief that germs are by far the most significant causes of all disease caused medicine to become primarily focused on treating the symptom rather than the whole person. Lifestyle and environmental factors were mainly ignored. The patients became mere observers of their treatment: handing responsibility for their health over to their doctors.

Pasteur's concept was later proved wrong and replaced by a new theory which postulates that it is the milieu, the environment, that is the main cause for disease to develop. Therefore, by changing the milieu, the bacteria have a reduced impact and healing can take place.

Proponents of Western orthodox medicine are restricted to the only tools available to them which consist of suppressing, cutting, dissecting, irradiating and poisoning.

This is fully in tune with the Newtonian view that human beings are three-dimensional machines with a computer on top which can easily be dealt with by repairing the faulty part, the symptom.

In recent years the demand for natural remedies and treatments has grown enormously. This reveals people's innate desire to work in alignment with nature to cure their ailments, giving hope that the ancients' knowledge will survive and remain available for generations to come.

In dentistry we can make use of natural remedies by incorporating essential oils into the patient's treatment. They are safe to use and are beneficial for their detoxifying, antibacterial, antiviral, immune boosting, pain relieving, anxiety reducing and calming properties. As an example, clove oil is beneficial in the relief of toothache.

Other natural remedies include flower formulas, Bach Flower Remedies, phytobiophysics, Australian bush flowers or gem, crystal and mineral essences, which all act as energy harmonisers, supporting the body to restore its physical, emotional and spiritual balance.

Alternatively, homeopathic remedies are highly-diluted substances made from plants, mineral, chemical or animal sources and are used with the purpose of triggering the body's self-healing mechanism.

In dentistry, homeopathic remedies have a huge range of applications. Some common ones being:

- Arnica to help with pain and swelling
- Symphytum and Hypericum to support bone healing after surgery
- Ledum to reduce the pain resulting from injections

If you are not looking after your teeth, your whole being including your emotions, mind and spirit may suffer.

The cutting-edge Light-Kinesiology method may also prove useful in your own healing journey.

Taking a holistic approach and moving towards the understanding that we are perfect the way we are, and that Mother Nature does not make mistakes, we come to understand that we create our own health and our teeth are an integrated part of this ecosystem.

SOLUTIONS AND TREATMENTS

You now have a deep awareness of the threats to your dental health and overall well-being. It is time to explore the various solutions that will allow you to develop your own effective approach to healthy and happy teeth, and beyond!

1. Genetics

The good news is you can change your health!

No matter how toxic dentistry may have affected you in the past, you can recover your health. There are steps you can take right now to help yourself and there are many dentists out there who are willing to help you with the health challenges that present themselves in your mouth.

You probably have heard someone saying, "I have the same teeth as my dad and his dad before. It's in the family, it's in the genes, you know."

It is true to say that we all inherit our genes from our parents. However, our genes are not our destiny, they merely load the gun. It is our environment, our epigenetics and our mental, emotional and physical state that pulls the trigger.

Current research suggests we will soon be able to grow our own new teeth, making a visit to the dentist a far less traumatic experience. Where dentists merely remove a defective tooth and plant the seed for a new one. Imagine the possibilities!

During the early 1900s, Dr. Weston Price conducted valuable research into the dental health of remote tribes all over the world. This included indigenous Africans, Australian aborigines, New Zealand Maori, Indians of North and South America, the Innuit and Native North Americans, Melanesian and Polynesian South Sea Islanders, tribes of Switzerland and the Outer Hebrides.

He discovered that because these tribes had very little contact with the Western world and its food supply, they very rarely suffered from tooth decay, gum infection, narrow dental arches or airway pathways or any kind of chronic disease. They were living according to the rules of nature.

Once in contact with the Western world's diet they very rapidly began to suffer from tooth decay and gum disease. Their offspring also developed narrower jawbones with crowded teeth and reduced immunity to disease. However, upon returning to their ancestral diet these diseases disappeared and after two generations even the narrow arches were gone.

This is evidence that, with the correct diet, we are in charge of our own well-being and can change our health for the better. We can therefore no longer blame our ancestors for our genes and our state of health. It is our responsibility to do whatever is necessary to keep our mind, body and spirit in good shape.

2. Diagnostics

In order to get to the root cause of your dental problem a thorough initial consultation is necessary. A holistic dentist's examination may therefore be more extensive than your normal check-up.

A holistic dentist integrates and applies conventional and alternative approaches to your dental health, is open to new therapies and most importantly, walks their talk.

They will check your medical history, teeth, gums, soft tissues, temporomandibular joint, and take X-rays or a 3D-scan if necessary. As well as discussing your dental hygiene regime a holistic dentist may perform other checks and tests such as:

- Your saliva and urine pH to establish your alkaline-acidity level
- An ultrasound scan (Cavitat™, Cavitau™) of your

jawbones, if an infection is suspected
- Your root canal and dead teeth for toxicity and for any gum infection using the OroTox™ Test
- Your plaque under a microscope
- An infrared thermographic picture of different areas of your face to look for differences in temperature which may show infections in your jawbones
- An electric current in your mouth
- Oral galvanism, if you have different metals in your mouth
- If mercury vapour is released from your amalgam fillings
- An adrenaline-free anaesthetic (Procain) into your gum over a suspected area, discovered on X-ray, ultrasound or 3D-scan, to see if there is a response such as pain reduction, which indicates a problem area
- An autonomic response test (ART), applied kinesiology (AK) or a bioresonance machine to get more information about your dental and overall health
- Your tonsils
- Your sinuses
- Your tongue for coloration, fissures, indentations and coating
- Your airways
- Your wisdom teeth, even if they are not impacted, because they can pose significant health problems
- Your symptoms and the tooth-body chart
- Your posture
- Further blood, hair, stool or urine tests e.g.
- compatibility of dental materials

- heavy metal burden
- The influence of your diet, supplement protocol and life style choices
- The benefits and risks of root canals and jawbone infections in relation to the tooth-body-connection

Each dentist has their own protocol for initial consultations. Therefore, this list is by no means exhaustive, however it gives you an idea of what to expect.

A word about X-rays: no one likes them and they should definitely be kept to a minimum (digital X-rays should be used to minimise radiation). However, they are absolutely essential for properly diagnosing your teeth, jawbones, TMJ, nerve pathway and sinuses.

Overall, you should trust your dentist, feel comfortable with them and be happy to ask any questions you may have. Having a good relationship with your dentist plays an important part in your healing process.

3. Treatment Preparation

Here are some helpful recommendations that you can use prior to treatment.

If your treatment involves the removal of amalgam fillings, you need to make sure that prior to the amalgam's removal you minimise the amount of mercury that is released from those fillings.

What you can DO to prepare for removal of amalgam fillings:

- Support your body with a balanced diet high in antioxidants
- Use a manual soft toothbrush and a non-abrasive toothpaste
- Brush your amalgam fillings only lightly
- Eat food high in sulphur such as bananas, parsley, kale, watercress, garlic, onions, avocado, beef, chicken, fish, lentils, because mercury depletes you of sulphur

In addition:

- Add supplements to your diet. Ideally natural ones or increase foods that are naturally high in these vitamins and minerals. These include glutathione, magnesium, methionine, selenium, vitamin B6, C, D3 and zinc
- Raise your saliva pH to around 7 where possible. This you can do by having a more balanced and alkaline diet, adding supplements, exercising gently and reducing your stress level

Best to avoid or minimise:

- Chewing gum, because it releases 50% more mercury than if you don't chew gum
- Grinding and clenching your teeth. If you grind your teeth, have your dentist make a soft tooth guard to wear at night, when most of the grinding takes place
- Electric and ultrasound toothbrushes because they release more mercury from the fillings than manual brushes due to their bristles being harder and touching the fillings more frequently

- Having an MRI-scan (especially the latest more powerful ones). New research indicates higher leakage of mercury from amalgam fillings due to the heat developed during scanning
- Consuming sugar, artificial sweeteners, fruit juices, alcohol and caffeine as this lowers your pH
- Wi-Fi
- Proximity to microwaves

4. HOLISTIC TREATMENT

If we look back, we can see that Western medicine is a very young discipline compared to the ancient Egyptian, Greek, Roman or Islamic approaches or indeed even the medicine of tribes like the Indigenous Australians or North Americans.

Ancient medicine used herbs, diet, acupuncture and had the knowledge of how to repair physical injuries. Rituals and prayers were also important elements in the healing process. This holistic approach evolved over time into allopathic medicine—resulting in doctors mainly looking at the symptoms and continued to expand into the unique specialisations we find in modern medicine today.

So, who looks at the whole patient? Who sees the bigger picture?

A holistic dentist looks at the whole patient and sees more than what is just going on in their mouth. The patient's oral health paints a picture of their overall health.

Imagine dis-ease as simply being your body showing you that an area of your life needs your attention. According to the famous German physician, Dr. Reinhard Voll, almost 80% of all illness is either entirely or partially related to problems within the mouth. With holistic dentistry we are moving beyond repair or mask medicine towards whole body dentistry, taking into account the patient's personal circumstances.

Now is the time to find yourself a holistic dentist.

There are several organisations such as the IAOMT (*International Academy of Oral Toxicology & Medicine*) and IABDM (*International Academy of Biological Dentistry and Medicine*) who can support you in finding the right dentist for you. Also check out relevant social media groups.

If you have to undergo any kind of dental treatment, it is of utmost importance that the procedures are performed with the best safety protocols available.

For example, the removal of amalgam fillings is best done by your dentist following the protocol of either IABDM or IAOMT. Removing your amalgam filling is likely to reduce your toxic load. However, it does not automatically cure all of your symptoms.

Surgical procedures, whether a tooth extraction or cleaning out an area of infected bone, require thorough cleaning out of the socket, removal of the periodontal ligament after extraction and scooping out any soft, infected bone. An application of ozone gas to eradicate bacteria and the placing of a membrane, made from your own blood, enhances the whole healing process and reduces bone recession.

Ideally, it would best to use an adrenaline-free anaesthetic to keep the blood flow as intact as possible during the entire process.

Treatments for gum disease can be greatly supported with laser, ozone and calcium therapy.

All patients benefit from a supplementation protocol before, during and after treatment, in order to optimise their body's healing and detoxification capacity.

Particular attention during treatment is given to providing high dosage vitamin C infusions to detoxify the body and reduce pain and swelling. An adequate VitD-3 level is important for proper healing.

Additional therapies like laser, magnetic field therapy, acupuncture, essential oils, herbal medicine, homeopathy, lymph massage, osteopathy, reflexology, Reiki or any other supporting healing therapy can greatly enhance the patient's recovery.

Research and the experience of dental practitioners show that the application of ozone gas can reverse tooth decay, gum disease, TMJ problems, mouth ulcers, cold sores and it can prevent root canal treatment by halting the decay infection from spreading into the pulp.

5. Detoxification

Detoxification is a way to rid your body of all sorts of toxins enabling the body to become healthier. It makes most sense and is far more successful and longer-lasting once all metals, toxins and infections are removed from the teeth and jawbones and the temporomandibular joints and the muscles are working in harmony.

There is a wide variety of detoxification methods available. Do-it-yourself methods you can easily adopt on your own and others which are guided by your health practitioner.

If you suffer from thyroid disease or *any* other medical condition, always consult your health practitioner before starting out on a detoxification protocol. You could do more harm than good, because to detox properly your liver and thyroid have to function well.

To detox properly you need a sufficient level of iodine for your thyroid to produce the hormones necessary to support the detoxification process. Therefore, your thyroid needs to be well saturated with iodine.

You can get a good idea if your body has a sufficient level of iodine by performing the iodine skin patch test.

Apply Lugol's Iodine solution in a concentration of 15% on the inside of your wrist, about 2x2cm square, and see how quickly the orange colour disappears. The more iodine-deficient you are the faster the colour disappears. If you are well saturated with iodine the colour should only start fading after about twenty to twenty-four hours.

A way of detoxing on the go is through intermittent fasting. Having dinner at 6pm then eating nothing until 12pm the next day, gives your intestines time to fully digest, allowing a more comprehensive internal cleansing process. This method is contrary to the belief that breakfast is the most important meal of the day.

Detoxification is a purification process that your body accomplishes on a daily basis to get rid of waste and toxins through the skin, liver, kidneys, lungs, lymph, blood, large intestine and kidneys.

From a dentist's perspective, one could argue that it is sufficient to get your dental toxins and infections out of your mouth and teeth. The question is whether this is enough to regain your health.

The toxins that made you sick in the first place are distributed throughout your body. Mercury, for example, accumulates amongst other organs in kidneys, intestine, spine, brain and in fat tissue. The toxins from infections prefer to accumulate in joints or muscle tissue.

Simply removing the toxic fillings will not be enough to remove the toxic load from those organs. Specific protocols have to be introduced and it has proven beneficial for a dentist to create a network of co-therapists who can assist and support the patient's detoxification process, to mobilise the toxins and eliminate them from the body.

Therefore, in order to detox properly these pathways must be open and working correctly to excrete the toxins from your body. Otherwise the toxins are removed from one area and redistributed to another.

Gentle ways to detox are detoxing foot baths and infrared saunas.

You can support your body in many different ways to make detoxification easier, including the use of high-dose intravenous vitamin C.

Detoxification protocols using chelation agents like DMSA, DMPS or EDTA are sometimes recommended. The application of these chelators can be challenging for the kidneys and the therapist must ensure that the interstitial tissue, where the exchange of nutrients and waste takes place, is unblocked at all times.

Patients have to be aware that a chelation protocol, due to the challenge it presents in measuring and replacing the correct balance of minerals, has to be closely monitored by their health practitioners.

Detoxification can take place on different levels.

You can detox on a physical level which includes blood, intestines, kidneys, liver, muscles and skin with methods such as lymph massage, exercise, deep breathing, bouncing on a mini trampoline, fasting, juicing, herbs, enemas, colonic irrigation, infrared sauna, body scrubs, foot baths, hot and cold showers, Epsom salt baths and infusion therapy to name a few.

You can also detox on a mental, emotional and spiritual level by releasing self-sabotaging behaviours, letting go of limiting beliefs, practising forgiveness and mindfulness, meditation, hypnosis, Light-Kinesiology, Neuro-Linguistic-Programming, Qi-Gong, EFT, Reiki, Time-Line Therapy or one of the many other treatments on offer.

A routine that greatly supports your detox effort is drinking half a litre of lukewarm water with a freshly squeezed lemon first thing in the morning.

During your detox program always picture the end result in your mind. Imagine emerging from it, knowing it was absolutely worth every single minute because you feel totally energised, inspired and rejuvenated.

6. Replacement Options

Here are the most commonly used non-metal options available to replace amalgam fillings, metal crowns or to fill the gap where teeth are missing.

Veneer: A veneer is a thin layer of ceramic placed over the surface of a tooth. It either improves the aesthetics of a tooth or protects a damaged tooth surface or straightens a misaligned tooth. It is made by a dental technician from an impression taken at the first visit. On the second visit it is cemented to the tooth.

Direct filling: A direct filling is where composite material is used for small to medium-sized cavities. They typically consist of a mixture of ceramic particles in plastic and come in many different variations. Although there are significant improvements being made to the content of composite fillings, there are still some which contain ingredients which are under investigation as being potentially harmful to human cells such as TEGMA, TEGDMA and Bis-GMA.

For sensitive patients, a test to establish which composite material is best for them may be recommended. Composite fillings shrink with age and may pull away from the tooth, allowing leakage.

Inlay: An inlay is an indirect filling made by a dental technician, which are mainly ceramic. Two visits to the dentist are needed. One to file the tooth and take an impression and the second to fit the inlay. Inlays normally last much longer than direct fillings and the tooth anatomy can be ideally copied.

Crown: A crown is needed when large parts of the tooth are damaged and can't be restored with a filling or an inlay. They cover the entire tooth. They too, are made by a technician, need two appointments and are made of ceramic, zirconia or zirconium oxide.

Bridge: A bridge is used to fill a gap with a false tooth where a tooth is missing in order to improve functionality and appearance. The procedure and materials are the same as with a crown, but at least two teeth have to be filed to fit the bridge.

The advantage of zirconium-oxide bridges is their high strength and high fracture toughness.

A bridge affects the intrinsic mobility of the teeth involved. It can also have a detrimental influence if the midline is crossed connecting a tooth from the left side of your mouth with a tooth on your right side. This is especially important in the upper jaw.

A speciality is the Maryland bridge, where the bridge wings on either side of the bridge are fitted on the palate side to natural teeth. This saves the teeth from being filed down like a crown.

Implant: A dental implant is an artificial root which is permanently placed in the jawbone to hold a false tooth in place. They are made of zirconia, zirconium-oxide or PEEK (a composite). Implants need to integrate with the bone to gain stability. Implants can hold crowns, bridges or dentures.

Implants are an alternative to bridges and partial dentures with the advantage that they do not put any load on surrounding teeth, as a bridge would do. There is no need to file any neighbouring teeth and they don't put pressure on the gum as dentures do.

Although implants are widely used they are not for everybody. Implants may not be an option for you if you suffer from a chronic condition, have poorly controlled diabetes or osteoporosis because the jaw may not heal properly and the implant may not fuse with the jawbone. Your oral hygiene must also be impeccable to maintain the implant and prevent infection around it.

However, I have experienced that even some healthy patients became ill after having zirconium implants placed.

Partial Denture: A partial denture is a removable appliance which replaces one or many teeth by holding on to some of the remaining teeth. They are normally made from acrylic.

Partial dentures are also available as flexible dentures made of materials such as nylon, which is very biocompatible. They are thinner, smaller and more comfortable to wear. These dentures can be made for just one side (unilateral) and with flexible clasps which put less stress on the teeth they are clasped to.

A new material for partial dentures is PEEK, which is less flexible and stronger than the ones made from nylon.

The recommendation is to get as much information as you can to make the decision that is right for you.

7. Oral Hygiene / Maintenance

Some families share them. Others use them for many months. Some don't use them at all. Toothbrushes.

The choice is yours as to which type you use. They come in a magnitude of different sizes, colours, shapes, strengths, bristles, handles and prices.

No matter what toothbrush you use, in order to optimise your oral health ensure that you clean every surface of every single tooth and in-between them. After cleaning your teeth, clean your toothbrush. You can do this by placing it in a 50:50 mixture of 6% hydrogen peroxide and water for five minutes and rinse well afterwards. This keeps bacteria at bay and your toothbrush fresh.

Surprisingly, toothpaste is not essential to clean your teeth. If you prefer to use one however, choose a brand without fluoride and other nasty chemicals which only disturb the finely tuned bacterial balance in your mouth.

You can also make your own toothpaste with sodium bicarbonate, sea salt and 3% hydrogen peroxide or use essential oils.

Blotting brushes don't require toothpaste and still leave teeth wonderfully smooth. They remove plaque from your teeth in the same way a painter blots excess paint from a canvas. This action also stimulates your energy pathways.

Ultrasound brushes can have a detrimental effect on the body (despite their cleaning effectiveness). Dr Wolfgang Burk's analysis of the use of ultrasound brushes revealed blockages similar to those in root canal-treated or dead teeth.

Summary: There are pros and cons to all of the options and materials. The choice you make will be dependent on parameters such as how many teeth are missing, how healthy are your gums, teeth and bone, your overall state of health, whether you prefer a fixed or a removable solution, aesthetic, phonetic and functional requirements and of course the price.

Cleaning your tongue with a tongue scraper to remove any plaque from your tongue also plays a vital part in your mouth's hygiene. This is especially important because the back part of your tongue can be a breeding ground for bacteria.

What you don't need is mouthwash, which can upset the natural bacterial balance in the mouth. If you use one, it should be all natural without alcohol. You can even use a few drops of essential oils, such as clove, peppermint or lemon mixed with water to freshen your breath.

Dental floss, tooth picks, interdental brushes and water picks are used to clean the areas in-between teeth. However, all these devices must be used diligently, otherwise they can do more harm than good. Research suggests that flossing has hardly any benefits and even the president of the *American Academy of Periodontology* acknowledged this.

Some experts say you are better off oil pulling. Oil pulling is performed by thoroughly swishing about a tablespoon of organic coconut oil through your teeth for round about 15 minutes. Then spit the oil into the bin and clean your teeth, tongue and cheeks of any remains.

The main intention of your oral hygiene regime is to remove the biofilm from your teeth, cheeks and tongue. The biofilm is the playground where the bacteria harbour. As long as you have a healthy diet and lifestyle your body is in a balanced state and the bacteria will do no harm.

Your body has more bacteria than human cells. And in your mouth alone there are about 100 to 200 different species.

Only 2% of people clean their mouth for more than a minute each time they brush. Congratulations if you do more.

However, even if you clean your mouth regularly and properly, you will have thousands of bacteria living on each tooth surface. Imagine how many will live there if you don't clean them thoroughly.

Having a healthy diet plays a major part in your oral hygiene regime. The less sugar and processed food you consume the easier it is to keep your teeth and gums healthy and the less likely it is that any detrimental effects like tooth decay or gum disease will occur.

8. Tooth-Body Connection

In the late 1940s, Dr. Reinhard Voll was able to demonstrate that Chinese acupuncture points really do exist. He documented a network of points resulting in energy pathways, called *meridians*.

These meridians connect specific teeth, organs, joints, sense organs, endocrine glands, spine, muscles, reflexes and emotions: connecting everything in your body. This integral connection means, if something happens in your mouth it will reflect in other parts of your body and may cause symptoms.

Therefore, because they can affect your whole body, it is really important that you look after your teeth. Almost 80% of all illness, according to Dr. Reinhard Voll's research, is at least partially related to problems in your mouth.

Luckily, more and more patients are becoming aware of these interconnections between different parts of their body.

Every single tooth is also connected to specific organs, joints, endocrine glands, muscles, spinal cord segments, sense organs and vertebrae.

When we begin to understand the concept of the tooth-body connection, it becomes clearer that a kidney problem could be triggered by a root canaled front tooth. The front teeth, kidneys, bladder and urogenital system are connected via the kidney meridian.

And as we have seen previously, root canal-treated teeth or dead teeth, as well as jawbone infections can prevent the flow of the meridians.

Now it also makes sense to remove a root canal-treated tooth to enable the energy to run smoothly again. Once this is done the kidney/urogenital problem can resolve, as has been seen many times by the author.

It is important to keep in mind these connections are not one-way streets. They work in both directions. This means a problem from your kidneys can affect the correlated front teeth.

Knowing about these connections can explain why your dentist sometimes might not find anything wrong with your tooth, despite you feeling to the contrary.

Many dentists, if they cannot find anything wrong and the patient's discomfort persists, will recommend a root canal treatment to switch off the pain. However, this may be just a symptomatic treatment whilst the root cause remains undiscovered.

As an example, if a tooth is decayed into the pulp, the orthodox way of looking at this problem is a root canal treatment. However, the question to ask is, why did the tooth decay in the first place, the answer to which will bring you to the real cause. This is most likely a pH imbalance due to lifestyle choices.

As you can see, the tooth-body connection offers a fascinating new perspective of looking at your teeth, your body and your overall health.

There is wisdom in your teeth!

9. KNOWLEDGE

Knowledge is key. You cannot know what you do not know and if you do not know, you do not look for it and therefore you cannot change what you do not know.

With knowledge you explore and learn things you never knew existed. When you stretch yourself and step out of your comfort zone, knowledge gives you the power to change your life.

You might not have heard of the toxicity of root canaled teeth or amalgam fillings. Therefore, when you have your dental treatment, you consent without questioning what your dentist is recommending, simply because you don't know any better.

If you have never heard of the tooth-body connection, you will not be looking for it. And even if you have, you might dismiss it as a load of baloney. It is as simple as that.

And whilst everyone is entitled to their opinion, there is a huge amount of research and anecdotal evidence to support everything that I have written in this book. Knowledge creates greater choice and once you have this knowledge you can make an informed decision regarding your dental treatment.

When it comes to your health and your teeth, it is important to have sufficient knowledge and understand what the proposed treatment is about. You have to be willing and able to ask questions such as:

- What options are available?
- What are the advantages and the disadvantages of each option?
- What are the risks?
- What are the benefits?

Additional questions you can ask your dentist are:

- What caused this?
- What would you do if you were me?

The internet offers a wealth of information and, whilst being very educational, it is still advisable to research the subject thoroughly. You will come across paid quacks and trolls discrediting alternative, holistic, integrative and even common-sense treatments, and vice versa.

It is important to do your own research, join groups on social media and keep asking questions.

Before long, you will gather enough information and develop a feeling for what is right for you. You will gain a sense of what is true and what or whom you can trust. If unsure you can always obtain a second opinion.

The more information and knowledge you gather, the more specific your questions will become until you know that you can make the right decision to optimize your dental health.

10. Mindset

It is hard to believe that most of our beliefs and values have already been imprinted within us by the time we are seven years old.

When our beliefs and values are being formed, we are finding our way in the world, we are discovering who we are and innocently believe everything we are told by our parents, peers and even teachers.

Furthermore, when we are between the ages of seven and fourteen, we are continuing to develop our own opinions, understanding more about ourselves and the world around us. Our mindset is therefore determined by our experience of the world.

We are continually being programmed and moulded by the world around us.

It is our core beliefs and values that form the deepest sense of who we are and the basis of our personality. Values are made up of those beliefs that have the most importance to us, which motivate us upfront and allow us to evaluate later. Beliefs however, are convictions that we trust as being true. They form the rules by which we run our lives, and which we will defend with our last dying breath.

You may ask, "What has this got to do with my health?" One could argue, "Everything!"

Because our mindset is the one thing that we are in control of, and despite being programmed by people and events around us, we still have the power to make our own conscious choices about our health.

We may have been fed the misconception that we alone cannot take responsibility for our health. However, we can, by gathering the right information.

Taking responsibility is similar to setting a goal.

Have you ever set a goal and achieved it? Yes, of course you have.

Have you ever set a goal and did not achieve it? I bet you did.

So, the question is not whether you can achieve your goals. The real question is "Why aren't you achieving your goals all of the time?"

You may or may not have noticed, you always have a reason, something along the lines of "wrong time, wrong place, too expensive, too sick, I cannot do anything about it, my kids, my husband, wife, dog, etc." All these reasons are simply excuses.

If you want to achieve your goals, and that means your health goals as well, you have to take responsibility for yourself and stop using excuses.

Reading this book will have given you the courage to take positive action towards recovering your health. You are not alone on this journey.

As an example, if you are planning on replacing your mercury amalgam fillings, you may want to ask yourself, "What do I want to achieve from getting this procedure done?"

Do you want to:

- Become free of toxins and heavy metals?
- Increase your energy?
- Reduce your allergic reaction?
- Improve your aesthetics?
- Decrease your headaches, anxiety or irritability?
- Clear the metallic taste out of your mouth?
- Improve your gut health?
- Increase your absorption of nutrients?
- Rid yourself of candida and muscle spasms?
- Improve your concentration and memory?

If you want to strive towards optimum health, goal setting is putting a marker in the sand that you can aim for. As you focus and move towards your goal you become even more motivated. And it is this motivation that drives you forward to achieve that goal and allows you to overcome the challenges along the way.

11. Spirituality

Spirituality is the pathway to inner freedom and enlightenment. It is being in touch with the human soul or spirit. It is a sense of being connected to something bigger than yourself with the aim of searching for, or understanding, the meaning of life.

Spirituality has to do with being mindful. This means being non-judgemental and aware of your thoughts and emotions. It is the self-regulation of attention with an attitude of curiosity, openness and acceptance.

Have you ever experienced moments of awe? Maybe whilst watching a stunning sunset, looking at the star-filled sky, connecting with nature, or even listening to your favourite piece of music. Have you noticed how time stands still and you are simply in the moment with life?

Spirituality opens you up to the bigger picture of existence, putting your day-to-day problems, such as tooth decay, into the perspective of a larger framework.

In order for us to function properly, our mind, body and spirit need to be in harmony.

In challenging times, when the outside world offers no satisfactory answers, people often feel the urge to turn their focus inwards and search for a solution inside of themselves. Focusing your thoughts inwards, you may discover completely different causes for your present circumstances. You may come into contact with your purpose, with your God connection or spirit, whatever you understand that to be.

Spirituality increases your inner growth and sense of peace. You may achieve a state of inner freedom and happiness, which allows you to be aware of, though no longer affected by, external forces. It may create a sense of deep connectedness with others and your environment each and every day of your life.

Meditation is useful to develop your sense of spirituality and there are many other techniques that support relaxation such as EFT, reiki, tai chi, visualisation, yoga, self-massage, self-hypnosis, qigong, deep breathing and muscle relaxation.

YOUR MOUTH, YOUR LIFE

Having come a long way, from the daunting and dangerous place where you experienced the darker side of dentistry, you have now arrived at a stronger, empowered and exciting place.

You understand the areas of life that influence your oral and overall health.

You have discovered inspirational ideas and impactful concepts to start or continue your transformational journey of well-being.

Now you are capable of moving beyond toxic dentistry.

Now you have information from the source.

Now you are equipped with practical knowledge.

Knowledge that goes way beyond traditional dentistry.

You now have the ability to:

- Make healthier life style choices.
- Deal effectively with the toxins that are all around you.
- Overcome your limiting beliefs and emotions and channel them into something inspiring
- Resolve any dental problems you may have.

You have invested in something much bigger than dentistry.

You have invested in the foundations of your health, happiness and well-being.

And your journey has only just started.

Now go for it. Do it. Use this book to help you.

And remember,

- Your teeth mirror your body
- Your teeth reflect your overall health
- Your teeth echo your emotions
- Your teeth show your relationship to your environment
- Your teeth are the link between your external and inner world

And there is so much more to discover, because

There is wisdom in your teeth!

FOR BONUS RESOURCES
AND TO EXPLORE THE RESEARCH
BEHIND THIS BOOK

SIGN UP:

www.
dentistry-transformed.com
/resources

ACKNOWLEDGEMENTS

This book could only have been brought about with the help of some amazing people.

The first to thank are my dear colleagues, Dr Graeme Munro-Hall and his wife Dr Lilian Munro-Hall, who wrote the book *Toxic Dentistry Exposed*. They are one of the early pioneers in holistic dentistry and I had the pleasure of working alongside them for many years in their UK clinic until they retired in 2017. Many of the extraordinary stories mentioned in this book were experienced in their clinic.

David Shephard, the genius NLP Master Trainer heading *The Performance Partnership*, who spent many hours and numerous occasions during training courses to introduce me to his book-writing secrets.

John Fielder, who supported me throughout the writing, helping me smooth the Germanisms and contributing valuable ideas.

All my amazing patients with their incredible stories. You have all encouraged me to get my message out so that even more people can benefit. As you took responsibility and left behind your traumatic experiences and toxic materials, you too were able to live healthy, infection and toxin-free lives.

Finally, my beloved Sam. With her outstanding skill set of being able to get into the reader's head, heart and beyond, she was capable of icing the cake by supporting me in making the stories still more gripping, entertaining and even the facts more interesting to read.

Dr Elmar Jung

Since qualifying as a dentist in the 1980s, Dr Elmar Jung has always advocated the value of holistic dentistry. Knowing that there is much more to dentistry than simply treating symptoms he embarked on a decades-long exploration of complementary diagnostic and treatment methods.

His additional qualifications include: a holistic dentist with the German Association of Holistic Dentists, a doctor of FX Mayr Medicine and a Heilpraktiker (German Naturopath).

After years of dental practice in Germany and at the prestigious Paracelsus Clinic in Switzerland, Elmar moved to the UK to work with the UK pioneers in holistic dentistry, Drs Graeme and Lilian Munro-Hall.

His first book (2012), Weapons of Plaque Destruction, with Graeme Dinnen, showed how to cure and prevent tooth decay and gum disease using the blotting technique and the incredible blotting brush.

Dr Elmar knows, first-hand, the damaging effects of poor nutrition and standard toxic dentistry in many, many patients. More significantly, he also knows the life-changing impact of his comprehensive metal-free treatments, detoxification and supplementation protocols and holistic approach.

Elmar's mission is to empower patients to take responsibility for their own health and well-being, shifting them from toxic dentistry to transformed dentistry.

Elmar now practices near Southampton and also lectures internationally. You can find out much more at:

www.dentistry-transformed.com/about

OTHER DotDotDot TITLES

Unconscious Incarceration
Gethin Jones
ISBN—978-1-907282-86-7
For those trapped in cycles of addictive behaviour, desperate to find a way out. A personal account of freedom and a guide for your own journey.

Domestic Abuse Rescue Essentials
Diana Onuma
ISBN—978-1-907282-92-8
For those whose need to leave overcomes the reasons to stay. How to claim your freedom, follow the exmplae of those who have gone before you and implement practical, effective strategies.

Breathe With Ease
Alison Waring
ISBN—978-1-907282-88-1
For those looking for a powerful, natural approach to health. How to enable those with asthma and other breathing-related challenges to breathe with ease.

The Little Book of Holistic Accounting
Emma J Perry
ISBN—978-1-907282-81-2
For those stuck in a job or path that is stifling. How to balance the books of your body, mind, heart and soul.

Lightning Source UK Ltd.
Milton Keynes UK
UKHW022008230521
384249UK00005B/141

9 781907 282911